D0247574

Clinical Supervision in Practice

12/04

UNIVERSITY OF
WOLVERHAMPTON
ENTERPRISE LTD.

Harrison Learning Centre
Wolverhampton Campus
University of Wolverhampton
St Peter's Square
Wolverhampton WV1 1RH
Telephone: 0845 408 1631

Telephone Renewals: 01902 321333
Please RETURN this item on or before the last date shown above.
Fines will be charged if items are returned late.
See tariff of fines displayed at the Counter. (L2)

Clinical Supervision in Practice

Some questions, answers and guidelines

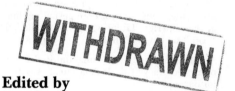

Edited by

Veronica Bishop

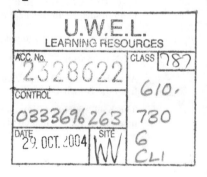

U.W.E.L.
LEARNING RESOURCES

ACC. No. 2328622

CLASS 787

610.

CONTROL 0333696263

730

DATE 29. OCT. 2004

SITE W

6 CLI

MACMILLAN

NTresearch

© This volume, *NT Research* and Veronica Bishop, 1998

© Selection, editorial matter, Preface, Chapters 1 and 2: Veronica Bishop, 1998

© Other chapters in order: Chris Maggs, Jeannette Davidson, Chrissy Dunn and Veronica Bishop, Nigel Northcott, Chris Scanlon, Jerome Carson, Anthony Butterworth, 1998

© Foreword: Yvonne Moores; Postscript: Susan Norman, 1998

All rights reserved. No reproduction, copy or transmission of this publication may be made without written permission.

No paragraph of this publication may be reproduced, copied or transmitted save with written permission or in accordance with the provisions of the Copyright, Designs and Patents Act 1988, or under the terms of any licence permitting limited copying issued by the Copyright Licensing Agency Limited, 90 Tottenham Court Road, London W1P 9HE.

Any person who does any unauthorised act in relation to this publication may be liable to criminal prosecution and civil claims for damages.

The authors have asserted their rights to be identified as the authors of this work in accordance with the Copyright, Designs and Patents Act 1988.

First published 1998 by
MACMILLAN PRESS LTD
Houndmills, Basingstoke, Hampshire RG21 6XS
and London
Companies and representatives throughout the world

ISBN 0–333–69626–3 paperback

A catalogue record for this book is available from the British Library.

This book is printed on paper suitable for recycling and made from fully managed and sustained forest sources.

10   9   8   7   6   5   4   3
07   06   05   04 03 02   01   00

Editing and origination by
Aardvark Editorial, Mendham, Suffolk

Printed in and bound in Great Britain by
Creative Print and Design Wales, Ebbw Vale

Contents

List of Figures, Tables and Boxes

Figures

Tables

Boxes

Foreword

The provision of health care has never been more complex. It demands multi-professional, multidisciplinary and multi-sectional communications and partnerships. As Professor Bishop identifies in her introductory chapter, the demands are for qualified nurses to be 'innovative, to develop new skills, to be answerable for their actions and to constantly update their knowledge'. Nurses and nursing face challenges to provide an evidence base to inform clinically effective practice, and to ensure the evolution of clinical practice and clinical roles.

I am convinced that clinical supervision has an important role to play and will be a key element in driving forward safe and innovative practice and will prove to be a fundamental way of supporting clinical colleagues at every level of the health service.

The importance of clinical supervision is that it maintains a focus on patient and carer needs and the quality of nursing practice. This is central to safeguarding standards, developing professional expertise and delivering quality care.

From the first discussions of clinical supervision in *Vision for the Future: A Strategy for Nursing, Midwifery and Health Visiting*, the concept has been taken forward in a variety of ways. Where successful as identified in the chapters written by Chrissy Dunn, Chris Maggs and Nigel Northcott, the important factor is that it is being driven by practitioners and reflects local needs and is set in the local context. It offers different things to different levels of nurse, novice or expert.

Clinical supervision is about constant refinement, broadening perspectives, and it is about enabling practitioners not controlling them. It requires time, the right and skilled supervisors. What has come across very strongly in our interactions with most sectors is that while clinical supervision must be part of the organisational structure, it must be owned by clinical nurses and not become unnecessarily bureaucratic.

To achieve successful and effective implementation clinical supervision requires something of a cultural change. We are not, as a profession, yet used to inviting critical debate. We are not good at sharing good practices nor are we always as skilled as we could be in constructively viewing less successful practice.

Clinical supervision is not common practice in all areas of nursing, in spite of the perceived benefits of enhanced practice for the benefit of patient care and the development of professional standards and personnel. Support for clinical leaders, particularly in flattened hierarchies, is seen as crucial to maintain and develop standards. Any such initiatives need to be set in tandem, and be supportive, to audit systems which are developed to ensure that patients, staff and their managers are achieving the maximum available to them.

What will work well in one environment may not work in another. Nurses working in rural areas may not have the same options as those in urban localities. Clinical supervision is not something that we can wave a wand over and the magical formula is there! We must get it right, it is so important, and we must be prepared to take it step by step.

The contributors to this book present individual perspectives ranging from theoretical concepts to practical application. What is demonstrated effectively is that clinical supervision is a 'dynamic process' that will improve health care and professional performance. I am sure that the reader will be fired with enthusiasm to commence and/or maintain the development of clinical supervision in their clinical environment.

Clinical supervision as part of a human resource strategy is not just a method of improving morale, recruitment and retention, but also a way to advance knowledge and practice.

YVONNE MOORES

Preface

This book is offered in the hope that it will convey the essential principles and aims of clinical supervision. Clinical supervision is not new across the health care disciplines, but there are many localities where it is being considered in a new dimension and, as such, the following chapters seek to offer guidelines and suggestions on how effective implementation of an important exercise may be achieved.

The individual contributors have voiced varied and different perspectives for the reader to consider, and, as is befitting in my view, I have not sought to blend their expert contributions into one homogenous style. Each contribution is unique, and I am most grateful to the authors for their support in producing what I hope will provide an interesting and very practical guide to implementing clinical supervision. I am also indebted to Linda Davidson and Jane Salvage of the *Nursing Times* for their support and help in contacting the Trust Nurse Executives involved in the text, and to the administrative staff of *Nursing Times Research*.

Clinical supervision must not founder for lack of initiative and ongoing support. Nurses, amongst others, need it to achieve their potential as individual and accountable practitioners offering the highest quality of services and care. Through this book, I hope to maintain commitment that I was fortunate enough to develop when the subject was new to many in the NHS. Clinical supervision is not an academic exercise, it is a dynamic process for practitioners. Don't take too long to read the book, this is a practical matter! Clinical supervision offers an opportunity not to be missed.

VERONICA BISHOP

List of contributors

Veronica Bishop SRN, FRSA, MPHIL, PHD

Editor of *NT Research*; visiting professor Anglia Polytechnic University; Health Care Consultant; previously lead Nursing Officer at the DoH for Clinical Supervision.

Tony Butterworth CBE, RGN, RNT, DN, RMN, MSc, PHD

Dean of School of Nursing, Midwifery and Health Visiting, Manchester University; Director for WHO Collaborating Centre for Nursing.

Jerome Carson BA(HONS), MSC, CPSYCHOL

Senior Lecturer in Clinical Psychology at Institute of Psychiatry, London; Honorary Consultant Clinical Psychologist with Bethlem and Maudsley NHS Trust.

Jeannette Davidson RGN, RM, DHSA DIPN, BA

Honorary Lecturer, Glasgow Caledonian University, Department of Nursing and Community Health; until September 1996, Nursing Officer holding the interest in Clinical Supervision at The Scottish Office Department of Health.

Chrissy Dunn RGN, DPSN, BSC(HONS)

Senior Practice Development Nurse, Royal Berkshire and Battle Hospitals NHS Trust.

Christopher Maggs SRN, FRSA, BA(HONS), MA, PHD

Professor of Nursing, University of Staffordshire; Director of R&D Mid Staffs General Hospital NHS Trust.

Nigel Northcott RGN, PGCEA, DɪpN, MA(Eᴅ), PʜD

Independent Nurse Consultant and Practitioner; former clinical leader of a Nursing Development Unit.

Chris Scanlon RN, RNT, CᴇʀᴛEᴅ(FE), DɪpHᴜᴍPsʏᴄʜ, MSᴄ

Lecturer/practitioner in psychosocial nursing, St Bartholomew's School of Nursing; specialist practitioner Royal London Hospital; tutor psychodynamic studies University of Oxford.

1

Clinical Supervision: What Is It?

Veronica Bishop

The professional and political reasons for the inclusion, as a high priority, of clinical supervision on the national nursing agenda are discussed and the main 'drivers' of current activity in clinical supervision explored. Various definitions of clinical supervision are offered, and the principles and ground rules necesssary for its effective implementation and anticipated outcomes are described.

Background

The emergence of clinical supervision as a major issue on the nursing agenda is an exciting development that offers the profession an opportunity to maximise its enormous potential both educationally and politically. It has been discussed and debated in nursing across all strata of the health care system since the early 1990s. Indeed, in several clinical specialties, such as mental health nursing, it has been practised in some localities and much valued by its users over many years. It was the Nursing Division at the Department of Health (DoH) that took the initial lead in placing clinical supervision as a priority agenda item for the profession.

The Allitt inquiry (Clothier report; Department of Health, 1994a) crystallised a number of concerns about the supervision and support of safe, accountable practice. On the same day in February 1992 that the Clothier report was published,

1

it was no coincidence that so also was a position paper on clinical supervision by Faugier and Butterworth (1994). This DoH-commissioned paper was distributed widely to the NHS, the professional bodies and the independent sector in England with an accompanying letter from the Chief Nursing Officer (DoH, 1994b), stating that she had no doubt as to the value of clinical supervision and considered it to be fundamental to safeguarding standards, to the development of professional expertise and to the delivery of quality care. The Position Paper was also distributed in Scotland, and the two countries were to liaise closely in setting the nursing agenda on clinical supervision. However, it should be emphasised that clinical supervision was not being promoted as a political sop for either bad publicity in nursing or low morale. The concept has been, and is being, promoted from within the profession because it is genuinely identified as, at worst, a mechanism to safeguard minimum clinical standards and public safety and, at best, a mechanism that will support the development of excellence in practice and thus high-quality nursing care. There are some cynics who regarded clinical supervision as a managerial stick and others who see it as a sop for low morale, but, in the light of how the concept is developing, these fears are, in the main, proving to be unfounded.

While the simultaneous distribution of the Clothier report (Department of Health, 1994a) and the Position Paper on clinical supervision was not coincidental, neither was it a coincidence that at meetings between the DoH, the professional bodies and practitioners across the country, the need for support while being innovative, the need to share good practices and the lack of interprofessional caring were raised. Data collected from over 2000 qualified nurses in England in a Delphi study (Butterworth, 1993) on what facilitated good practice voiced strong support for clinical supervision, this theme being extended into the much-debated and refined *Vision for the Future: The Nursing, Midwifery and Health Visiting Contribution to Health and Health Care* (DoH, 1993) and emerging as a specified target. Twelve targets were identified in this document for achievement over the following year, target 10, in particular, stating that:

discussions should be held on the range and appropriateness of models of clinical supervision.

Similarly, the Government's review on mental health nursing (DoH, 1994c), circulated a year later, was to support strongly the concept of clinical supervision.

So why the apparent sudden interest in this concept of professional support and peer review? Historically, it can be seen that the nursing profession gets an occasional 'bee in its bonnet' – the nursing process, for example – so what, if anything, is different now? Is this some ploy to control a large workforce, under the guise of professional develop-ment? That question has certainly been asked more than once. What is different now has several facets, not least the structure and organisation of the NHS. Flattened professional hierarchies have resulted in fewer opportunities to discuss work, and the increase in care in the community often means that nurses are isolated and missing the traditional peer support mechanisms, such as they were. There is often a feeling among clinical staff that is embodied in the phrase by Charles Handy (1994):

> if [economic] progress means that we have become anonymous cogs in some great machine, progress is an empty promise.

Frequent organisational changes, limited budgets set against high demand and high turnover, the introduction of an internal market system and the separation of services (and staff) are hardly conducive to high morale.

An excellent, unofficial discussion document (NHSE, 1992), prepared and circulated for regional consultative conferences on the then new English Strategy for Nursing (DoH 1993), contained highly pertinent and thought-provoking statements within the context of massive change, both in service demands and delivery, and in terms of nurse education and changing professional roles. Niall Dickson and Frances Pickersgill, the main authors, who are prominent in the nursing profession's ongoing debates, suggested that new ways to improve what happens between professionals and their patients and clients needed to be identified. They stated:

> neither nursing nor any of the health disciplines are ends in themselves and the task facing the health service must be to ensure that staff are able to do everything possible to maximise patient well-being not only by improving the care received by each individual... but also by ensuring that professionals and other staff are empowered to contribute to developments in the service and to help shape local policy.

This working document stressed the belief in a wealth of untapped potential in the nursing workforce; evidence of what can be achieved has surfaced in a host of practice developments as innovative practitioners have adapted patient care to meet changing needs and demands, as for example in the Nursing Development Unit (NDU) programme and nurse-led services, the tenets expressed holding good today and for the foreseeable future.

With such developments and the concomitant need for nurses to be accountable for their own practice, to be up to date on professional knowledge and to participate fully as a health team member comes the absolute necessity of professional critique and questioning. The obligation to question our practices, to seek review and to test and retest our values, which should be a part of any established discipline, is rarely, as yet, intrinsic to our nursing culture. Neither is the value of sharing our successes as well as our disappointments – but, to achieve true professionalism, this culture change has to happen.

The demands on qualified nurses to be innovative, to develop new skills, to be answerable for their actions and constantly to update their knowledge were initially highlighted in the United Kingdom Central Council for Nursing, Midwifery and Health Visiting (UKCC) guidelines on professional accountability (UKCC, 1992), which stated that the practitioner:

> must act in a manner so as to promote and safeguard the interests and well-being of patients and clients, maintainand improve professional knowledge and competence.

The introduction of post-registration education and practice (PREP) (UKCC, 1995) should be seen as helpful to this process.

However, this will only work where nurses are willing to accept full accountability for their own practice and can feel confident enough to challenge systems and procedures which undermine good practice.

The nursing profession has the responsibility of self-regulation: those nurses who do not uphold the standards laid down can be removed from the professional register, and considerable time is spent regulating those who transgress the rules. It is ironic, however, how little time is spent on developing systems to sustain practice and offer protection to service users and professionals. Extended clinical practice, increased autonomy and a greater degree of decision-making have combined to make the need for clinical supervision more obvious. Critchley reports that the supervisory process, when properly and responsibly carried out, can enhance nurses' abilities to observe, describe and understand more accurately, and to make fewer assumptions about their clients or their own behaviour (Critchley, 1987), findings supported by a small study carried out in Finland (Paunonen, 1991).

A purchaser's perspective (Bishop and Butterworth, 1994) has highlighted the 'explosion' of practice nursing over the past few years and the major proliferation in that area, with some excellent practice development. However, with this development comes the drawback of isolated working for many of our colleagues. Such a growth in practice may also put people in pressurised situations, with the potential to compromise on standards. Similarly, the increase in the number of private nursing homes to meet the needs of continuing care in the community for the mentally ill and those with learning disabilities may put nurses in unsupported and critique-free environments, thus jeopardising professional growth and skill development. Health visitors are another group put under particular strain, not least with changes in the law pertaining to child protection. Many models of clinical supervision amongst health visitors have developed out of the necessity to support staff solely in this area of work and are now being developed further to accommodate all areas of the health visitor's role.

There is much anecdotal evidence to suggest that the increased activity in all areas of health care has put staff at grass-roots level – those who have the responsibility to maintain standards of care – under incredible stress. Clinical supervision must come into its own here; it must be presented as it is intended to be – therapeutic, 'something for nurses', not a disciplinary or critical event. However, not having a system of clinical supervision in place which enables staff to reflect on their practice may well be considered unsound by future official judges of health care delivery, as it was by Clothier, and pertinent to this particular debate is the Health Service Commissioner's report (Wilson report; DoH, 1994d) and the devolution of complaints procedures to NHS Trusts rather than through the Department of Health. The case for sharing good practices, and minimising if not eradicating anything less than quality care, is clearly spelled out in the Wilson report. Clinical supervision, if implemented sensibly, will be a powerful tool in achieving this. A key to its success lies in allowing practitioners to own it, rather than to 'power drive' it from the top, an issue on which the Trust Nurse Executives were all agreed in their early discussions.

Of particular importance in taking the concept of clinical supervision forward in England and turning it into a reality were the meetings between the Chief Nursing Officer for England and her Trust Nurse Executive colleagues. The other UK countries developed similarly, sometimes ahead, sometimes in tandem, the aim always being to share and develop a solid approach to support nursing. The topic was always high on the agenda, and, like Topsy, it grew, flourishing as its potential importance for the profession became clearer. What was not so clear, however, were the agreed fundamental elements that needed to be embedded in any definition of clinical supervision, nor the 'how' of taking clinical supervision forward. Three years on, these issues are, as yet, still unrefined but are undergoing careful consideration and experimentation. The debate at these early meetings led to the organisation of workshops, seminars and conferences, not only in England, but also collaboratively with Scotland. However, the rest of the UK was not losing time, and in Wales clinical supervision was perceived as an important development, with the potential to improve patient care and was, as such, linked with the national clinical effectiveness initiative. Similarly, a number of initiatives have been taken forward in Northern Ireland since the Chief Nursing

Officer issued a professional letter and guidance to the Health and Social Services in 1994. Here it was recognised that clinical supervision had a central role to play in supporting the development of innovation in practice that is systematically evaluated and assessed. Local guidance has since been produced, and, in a number of Trusts, lines of professional supervision have been set up to ensure that individuals working within multidisciplinary clinical teams have access to personal support to safeguard standards and develop professional expertise. Across the UK, the issues raised and the degree of consensus achieved are as described below.

Semantics: a working definition

The debate on the subject was, not surprisingly, both enriched and confused by opposing and complementary points of view. Nursing already had 'mentorship' and 'preceptorship'; did it need anything else? What was different about clinical supervision? And who wanted 'supervision' anyway in an accountable profession? The connotations of the term 'clinical supervision' were not good, redolent as they were of task-oriented mentality, authority and control over the qualified practitioner. What is important about the terminology is that the focus is on clinical practice – the heart of what nursing is about – and it describes a mechanism to support the best in clinical developments. Despite the semantics (an issue that the UKCC is mindful to change, in time), those who had experienced ongoing clinical supervision were convinced of its importance to practice. However, its implementation is not yet the norm, and the models used vary to such an extent that to compare the value of one model with another presents enormous difficulties in terms of measuring value judgements, cost-effectiveness and clinical outcomes. This lack of clarity is slightly resolved by the findings from the DoH-funded study of 23 clinical supervision sites across England and Scotland (Butterworth *et al.*, 1997). However confusion was, and still is to a degree, exacerbated by the existence of a largely more generally managerial model of supervision that is a statutory requirement for practising midwives and has been used to some degree by social workers. It should be noted that, while this publication does not seek to address midwifery supervision, midwives are currently reconsidering their model in use.

To ensure that everyone involved in discussions shares the same interpretation of the term 'clinical supervision', a working definition (Faugier and Butterworth, 1994) has been widely used:

> an exchange between practising professionals to enable the development of professional skills, an opportunity to sustain and develop professional practice.

Thus while the terminology may be disputed, the concept is not.

The following definition (Hart, 1982) is similar:

> an ongoing educational process in which one person in the role of supervisor helps another person in the role of supervisee to acquire appropriate professional behaviour through examination of the supervisee's professional activities.

More recently, I have adopted the definition agreed at workshops held at Anglia Polytechnic University:

> Clinical supervision is a designated interaction between two or more practitioners, within a safe/supportive environment, which enables a continuum of reflective, critical analysis of care, to ensure quality patient services.

For me, the essential components of the adapted Proctor (1992) model are enshrined in this definition, which highlights the necessary key issues – protected time, confidentiality, research-based practice, shared expertise and staff empowerment.

Trust Nurse Executives have provided the toughest and most influential material for the development of clinical supervision. At workshops (DoH, 1994e) with the Trust nurses, and at a national conference (Bishop and Butterworth, 1994) open to all levels of nursing staff, the issues were debated until a degree of consensus was obtained on basic principles. In brief, the conference consensus statement endorsed the need for clinical supervision to be developed and evaluated throughout the health service. The need was identified for flexible models to be implemented that met local needs. This was seen as offering a potentially significant contribution to the provision of safe practice, quality care and accountable practice. Clinical supervision was seen as an effective way to help purchasers and providers access the experience and expertise of nurses through discussing and sharing practice development. It was also seen as a method that professionals could use to sustain and develop practice in a manner receptive to changing needs. These principles were later adopted by the UKCC in its statement on clinical supervision (UKCC, 1996) and hold good today. So what were the agreed principles?

Functions of clinical supervision

Clinical supervision was not regarded as camouflage to hide hierarchical domination. It was agreed that clinical supervision was about empowerment rather than control and that it demanded both time and investment. Indeed, properly carried out clinical supervision was not seen as a cheap option but, in the view of some, one with a heavy price. However, into the financial equation must also go the costs of litigation, of the loss of unmotivated, qualified staff and of poorer quality care than could be achieved.

The Trust nurses considered that clinical supervision should be a part of the organisational structure but stated that it was essential for it to be owned by clinical nurses and avoid becoming stifled by unnecessary bureaucracy. They considered that a model of clinical supervision addressing formative, normative and restorative functions, as described and adapted from Proctor (1992) had both value and merit. These functions are well documented elsewhere (Butterworth and Faugier, 1992; Hawkins and Shohet, 1992; Butterworth, 1996) and may be abbreviated into developmental needs (formative), an opportunity for de-stressing and recharging (restorative), and professional monitoring (normative). It is helpful to consider these components separately, as, while the amount of time spent on each may vary according to the needs of the supervisee, each is likely to arise in some measure.

Formative function (educative/developmental)

Developmental needs may be met by knowledgeable support while the supervisee is undertaking a course or a degree, by advice on reading material or by the identification of a willing expert in a particular field. For those embedded in clinical work, action learning may be exceptionally beneficial as it offers the opportunity for shared experiences that is intrinsic to clinical supervision. This method of learning is well described by Revans (1976), who believes that effective learning really begins only when people have the opportunity constructively to share their difficulties, concerns and experiences with others. Reflective learning has been a part of the NDU culture (discussed in Chapter 6) and has been further developed, particularly by Christopher Johns (1995), who leans heavily on the psychodynamic model. Certainly, our preoccupation with formal methods of knowledge has led to a neglect of other, more personal learning methods – that almost osmotic effect of conferring with or observing an experienced and knowledgeable practitioner.

Restorative function (debriefing/recharging)

The restorative element – that part which supports professionals to unload their stress, in effect to 'debrief' – is central to clinical supervision. Nursing does not have a good history of taking care of its own; indeed, the current NHS 'macho' style of management has created its own culture of depersonalisation, which has permeated the profession in its striving for managerial and professional equality. Benner and Wrubel (1989) exquisitely describe 'burnout', finding it to be a peculiarly modern mistake to think that caring is the cause of burnout and that the cure is to protect oneself from caring in order to prevent the problem. They consider that loss of caring is the sickness and that the sufferer needs to be reconnected to sustain relationships, thus overcoming the alienation of burnout. It may sometimes be a fine line between the reconnection described here and the 'tea break, tear break' warned of by Butterworth

(Butterworth and Faugier, 1992); it will fall to supervisors to keep the balance between constructive and negative de-stressing.

Normative function (standard-setting/monitoring)

In considering the normative processes of clinical supervision, much debate has centred around the tension that may occur between management control and professional interests. Marinker (1994) found that paradoxes are not always opposites but rather competing goods, a view subscribed to by Handy, who describes paradoxes as the co-existence of simultaneous opposites and believes that they do not have to be resolved but rather managed (Handy, 1994). This is easy to say but not necessarily without its implementation difficulties. The UKCC has spent considerable time considering this, among other issues on clinical supervision, and has arrived at a generally acceptable philosophy in which it is acknowledged that, while links between individual performance review (IPR) and clinical supervision will inevitably occur, IPR cannot be used as a substitute for clinical supervision and any involvement of IPR processes should only be at the request of the practitioner (Darley, 1995). Proctor emphasises the need for clear working agreements for supervision alliances, with clarity of task and intent within the employing organisation, and clear and specific agreed boundaries of information and confidentiality between supervisor, practitioner and managers (Proctor, 1992). I find the components of the normative element that are highlighted in Figure 1.1 to be particularly helpful in considering what is meant by 'normative'. The emphasis on standard-setting and professional issues link, as they must, with management, but the overall activity is predominately professionally driven. Buttigeig (1995) considers that clinical supervision will benefit the nursing professions only if it is seen as part of the fabric of the organisation and stresses that, in her view, management supervision and clinical supervision are different functions and should not be undertaken by the same individual. She goes on to state that the functions are separate but complementary, which must be understood throughout the organisation.

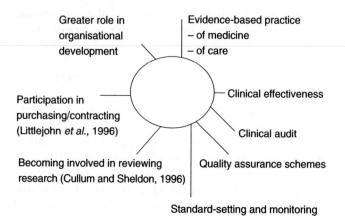

Figure 1.1   The normative functions of clinical supervision (adapted from van Ooijen, 1996)

Goals of clinical supervision

So if clinical supervision is not about control and is not a managerial tool, what are its goals? Platt-Koch (1986) describes them as the expansion of the practitioner's knowledge base, assisting in the development of professional autonomy and the growth of autonomy and self-esteem as a professional. Much has been written about the aims of clinical supervision (Butterworth and Faugier, 1992; Faugier and Butterworth, 1994; Butterworth *et al.*, 1996a) and these are well expressed. However, for convenience and without losing the heart of the matter, these may be condensed or simplified into three overall aims:

- to safeguard standards of practice;
- to develop the individual both professionally and personally;
- to promote excellence in health care.

In a guest editorial on the vital role of clinical supervision in clinical risk management, the UKCC's Chief Executive/Registrar (Norman, 1997) wrote:

the framework of the clinical supervision model gives nurses the opportunity to audit the quality of their practice through reflection. It enables nurses to identify and overcome shortcomings in practice, encourages that practice to be research based... with the result that standards are maintained and the potential harm to the patient is minimised – an obvious risk management tool.

It is important to identify the expectations, quality control and feedback mechanisms of any model (Bishop, 1994), and there are ground rules for clinical supervision if these goals are to be attained. The slogan 'A dog is for life, not just for Christmas' holds good for clinical supervision – it is not for a week, a month or even just while this or that innovation is going on, but for an entire professional life. This means that the time and accompanying resources must be protected.

Organisation of clinical supervision

How are we going to manage it? How do you eat an elephant? A bite at a time. (Bishop and Butterworth, 1994, p. 17)

Kohner (1994), in her study of some of the NDUs in which clinical supervision was implemented, and Butterworth (Butterworth *et al.*, 1996b) in his review of the literature and from initial findings of a multisite DoH study undertaken at Manchester University, have identified similar organisational requirements essential for the successful implementation of clinical supervision. These bear out the early statements made by the Trust Nurse Executives (DoH, 1994e) and may be listed accordingly:

- managerial commitment at every level;
- protected resources in terms of time, budget, manpower and training;
- supervision for supervisors;
- the establishment of evaluation techniques;
- the application of evaluation data to service management.

Managers vary in their views on the cost of clinical supervision. Much depends on how current resources are used in terms of staff education budgets, the use of agency staff, staff turnover, sickness levels and quality control/litigation. As data become available from Trusts, and as mechanisms for contracting that include clinical supervision develop, realistic costings will evolve. The view held by Nicklin, following his research findings (Nicklin, 1997), is that nurses are contributing, or are owed, £50 million unpaid overtime (the estimated cost of implementing clinical supervision). However, current uncertainty of hard costing and concrete gains puts the onus on our professional leaders to drive clinical supervision ahead with little of today's currency – something of an act of faith when faced with hard-nosed cynicism. Yet the other side of this debate is the shocked surprise voiced by some managers from other disciplines who had presumed such a mechanism already existed to ensure advanced and safe practice.

Costs will obviously vary according to the model of clinical supervision used and the time allocated to it. For example, one-to-one sessions will cost more than group sessions in the short term, but the group method may be less effective for some individuals. Network supervision, by Internet systems, telephone or even post, is an option that has to be developed for those in very isolated areas, if only on a maintenance level, and will cost little after the initial outlay.

Whichever model is used, with whatever time allocation, it is important that it is specific to the health care setting and is flexible within prescribed criteria. A Chief Executive, in his presentation to the DoH-funded national conference in Birmingham (Bishop and Butterworth, 1994), stated that one of the major points about clinical supervision was, in his view, that it is about utilising the resource of people in the organisation to their best advantage. Every member of staff in every part of the health care organisation needs time to improve practice; this is not a cost but an investment. It is certainly a view taken by Ashworth Special Hospital, where a 2-day skills course for clinical supervision was set up in 1995. The hospital is now developing minimum standards focusing on contract agreements between supervisee and supervisors, minimum standards for the frequency and duration of sessions, and training for supervisors.

Many current models of clinical supervision are run on the basis of one-to-one supervision for 1 hour each month. Brief, agreed notes are usually kept by both the supervisor and the supervisee as an *aide-mémoire* for the next meeting, and reflective diaries are sometimes kept by supervisees. The legal status of reflective diaries is not without concern, and those using this method of reflective learning should be aware that such documents, however personal, could be called into use in legal circumstances. Any model will have the informal and formal elements described by Faugier and Butterworth (1994) and should be negotiated by all staff, particularly if a multidisciplinary approach is used. Everitt (1996) describes an example of a clinical supervision contract that takes into account the type of supervision agreed, its theoretical orientation and the boundaries and documentation of sessions, as well as issues of structure, confidentiality and (subjective) evaluation. The importance of contracting between supervisors and supervisees is an important issue in implementing clinical supervision – it should provide the 'let out' clause for unworkable relationships, as well as the marker for those variables which may be audited, for example the frequency and duration of meetings.

Discussions with practitioners across England and Scotland have led me to believe that there is, as yet, not much enthusiasm for multidisciplinary supervision. Indeed, at this stage, a preference prevails for unidisciplinary models, although analysis of the questionnaire sent to Trust Nurse Executives (see Chapter 2) shows some move to multidisciplinary involvement. We are at the beginning of a long and potentially fruitful journey, and no options should be left unconsidered. It is helpful to be able to identify clearly the specific nursing role in any environment, but this must be undertaken in the wider context of the health care team. One thing is certain: while clinical supervision is, at the moment, a high-profile issue in nursing, recently further endorsed as such with the allocation, by Secretary of State for Health of the then-elected Conservative Government, of funding specifically for this purpose (DoH, 1997), the cultural shift required to make it successful will extend out to other professions, some of whom have long embraced the concept.

Butterworth and Bishop, with the NHS Executive (NHSE) and *Nursing Times* colleagues, have considered how best to present the concepts of clinical supervision to those seeking

advice and information. It was seen as important to emphasise the responsibilities and rights that must be in place in any
model used so that users of the guidance would not under-
estimate the issues involved. These have been very helpfully
provided with other useful background and reference information in the NHSE resource pack, *Clinical Supervision – a
Resource Pack*, currently available from the Nursing Directorate
of the NHSE, Leeds.

Selection and skills of supervisors

The importance of the role of the supervisor cannot be overestimated if effective clinical supervision is to be practised.
There are three types of credibility required by the supervisor in order to achieve effective clinical supervision: personal,
organisational and clinical. Any training of supervisors will need
to consider the development of facilitative skills, the management of personal and professional boundaries, and the need
for good listening and communication skills. The supervisor
must establish a safe environment, adhering to the agreed
rules on confidentiality. It should be noted, however, that it
is a statutory requirement for misconduct to be reported
(UKCC, 1992), and this must be recognised in the agreed
pact on confidentiality. Supervisors must confront their
personal and professional blocks, and the discussion must be
practice led. Critical to successful supervision is the identification of the issues to be discussed. Supervision sessions are
at first sometimes strained, and it may be helpful initially to
discuss case loads in order to identify the issues to be addressed.
Supervisees may find difficulty in sharing doubts and anxieties; crucial for progress is a contract between supervisor and
supervisee highlighting in particular the need for confidentiality. To be challenging while maintaining a positive approach
is not always easy, but good supervisors must achieve this if
supervisees are to benefit from sessions and be open to feedback, be willing to question their practices and explore new
interventions. This entire process is more likely to have the
desired outcomes if the supervisee has had some choice in
the selection of the supervisor.

Fowler (1995) has identified, through focus group discussion, that nurses' perceptions of good supervision can be grouped into three themes: relevant knowledge, supervisory/teaching skills and personal relationship skills. Certainly, the selection and training of supervisors is an issue that requires careful attention and has been the main thrust of the work on clinical supervision taken forward in Wales. Feeding into the Welsh Office NHS Trust initiatives is the work of Rafferty and Coleman (1996), who have designed educational preparation for clinical supervision that is organised to offer consistent theoretical and philosophical perspectives, experiential opportunities to engage in supervisory relationships and processes, with exposure to a range of organisational issues and ground rules. Discussions with many practitioners, acting in the capacity of either supervisor or supervisee, confirm my view that supervisors must be trained and supported; they must guide, rather than control or judge, and must follow the 'CCIS' principle – **C**hallenge, be a **C**atalyst, **I**nform and **S**upport.

Perceived benefits of clinical supervision

The perceived benefits of clinical supervision are well described by Kohner (1994), who studied five DoH-funded NDUs. The benefits include enhanced patient care, professional growth with self-assurance and confidence, broadened thinking and improved relationships between all parties in the health care scenario. The role of the King's Fund Centre in supporting the work of the NDUs cannot be overestimated, as the project team has brought education and support to the clinical areas involved.

Educationalists are, at last, beginning to understand that education is about adapting to the needs of the individual instead of pressing the individual between the leaves of conventional learning. Changing attitudes to learning, and changing perceptions of patient and clients, have put nurses in a strong position to bring the best to health care. Patients and clients have, overall, a greater understanding of their needs, and nurses are contributing in a major way to making sure that access is available. Nurses are taking on new roles: bridging the gap between education and practice with joint partnerships, meeting challenges with an enthusiasm that, in the main, harnesses enormous power for the good of health care. However, enthusiasm without skill enhancement, innovation without safety, energy without sustenance, will all result in lost promise and disillusionment. For the benefits of clinical supervision to be realised, quality and caring must count within the profession which is directed to itself.

At the hospital where I trained, I was asked recently 'If you were to walk onto a clinical area, what would be the key indicators that clinical supervision was received in that area?' The more experienced readers know where they would not wish to be cared for within moments of a visit, as good care can be recognised in an instant. This instinct is developed through specific knowledge and the combination of professional and lived experience; it is not achieved through theory alone, but is enhanced learning through action. It will not be easy to determine an objective measure to identify the effects of sharing those attributes with colleagues, and an even greater challenge lies in linking the benefits of clinical supervision with clinical outcomes. However, the importance of support, reflective and proactive thinking in driving clinical practice forward into excellence must not be underestimated while we search for adequate measuring devices and analytical methodologies to prove what the experienced amongst us know instinctively. The current buzzwords 'evidence-based practice' link logically with evidence-based supervision, and this must be the way forward in any planning. However, the difficulty of identifying all the components of nursing, as opposed to measuring the effect of discrete interventions, is far from resolved, and, while I would not wish to promote unthought-out actions in patient care, we cannot always wait for cast-iron proof. Little of what we do is based on such academic luxury anyway, so why be coy now? As an enthusiastic and committed Nigel Northcott informed a meeting which I was chairing, 'Why are you sitting here talking about it – you should be out there doing it!'

Conclusion

The recognition of the need for clinical supervision is wide-spread, as demonstrated by the tremendous commitment of Trust Nurse Executives to implement it despite their over-stretched resources and the many corporate demands on their agendas. Through their lead, and through the determination of their staff to provide the best care possible, we may yet achieve the culture change needed for us to grow into the strongest and most competent health care professionals. They are the brokers to instigate clinical supervision, and must negotiate to ensure the time, space and commitment essential to its effectiveness. Clinical supervision is, with its potential, a low- cost option offering enormous value for money. Literature on the subject is accumulating almost daily, and in some areas resource packs are being developed that are invaluable to guide those less travelled along this road. I am regularly approached for advice and information on clinical supervision by nurses undertaking dissertations and higher degrees or carrying out related research. Unless they all fall by the wayside – and their determination suggests that this will not be the case – we shall have a large body of knowledge within the next couple of years from which to pick the best, consider our position and strengthen our resolve. How the concept is 'sold' will vary according to available mechanisms, be it through clinical effectiveness, risk management, audit or other quality 'sound bites'. The tragedy will be if the sound aims of clinical supervision become an echoing rhetoric. Anthony Wedgewood Benn is attributed with the saying:

> There are kings and there are prophets. The kings have the power, the prophets have the principles.

There are, I believe, times when we all may have the opportunity to play either role professionally. In terms of health care services, the spelling of 'prophet' may need reconsideration, but of one principle I have no doubt – the power of clinical supervision – if it is managed responsibly.

References

Benner, P. and Wrubel, J. 1989 *Primacy of Caring*, Addison Wesley.

Bishop, V. 1994 Clinical supervision for an accountable profession. *Nursing Times* **90**(39): 34–9.

Bishop, V. and Butterworth, T. 1994 *NHSE Clinical Supervision Conference Proceedings*. London: NHSE.

Butterworth, T. 1993 *A Delphi Study of Optimum Practice in Nursing, Midwifery and Health Visiting*. Manchester: Manchester University.

Butterworth, T. 1996 Primary attempts at research-based evaluation of clinical supervision. *Nursing Times Research* **1**(2): 96–101.

Butterworth, C.A. and Faugier, J. 1992 *Clinical Supervision and Mentorship in Nursing*. London: Chapman & Hall.

Butterworth, C., Carson, J., White, E., Jeacock, J., Clements, A. and Bishop, V. 1996b *It's Good To Talk? The 23 Site Evaluation Project of Clinical Supervision in England and Scotland: an Interim Report*. Manchester: Manchester University.

Butterworth, T., Bishop, V. and Carson, J. 1996a First steps towards evaluating clinical supervision in nursing and health visiting. Part 1: Theory, policy and practice development. A review. *Journal of Clinical Nursing* **5**: 127–32.

Buttigeig, M. 1995 Foreword. In: *Clinical Supervision, the Principles and Process*. London: HVA.

Critchley, D.L. 1987 Clinical supervision as a learning tool for the therapist in milieu settings. *Journal of Psychological Nursing* **25**: 8.

Darley, M. 1995 *Nursing Management* **1**: 9.

Department of Health 1993 *Vision for the Future: The Nursing, Midwifery and Health Visiting Contribution to Health and Health Care*. London: HMSO.

Department of Health 1994a *The Allitt Inquiry. Independent Inquiry Relating to Deaths and Injuries on the Children's Ward at Grantham and Kesteven General Hospital during the Period February to April 1991* (Clothier report). London: HMSO.

Department of Health 1994b Clinical supervision for the nursing and health visiting professions. CNO Letter 94(5). London: HMSO.

Department of Health 1994c *Working in Partnership; A Collaborative Approach to Care. Report of the Government Review of Mental Health Nursing*. London: HMSO.

Department of Health 1994d *Report of the NHS Complaints Review Committee* (Wilson report). London: DoH.

Department of Health 1994e *Clinical Supervision: A Report of the Trust Nurse Executives' Workshops*. London: HMSO.

Department of Health 1997 Press Office Release.

Everitt, J. 1996 Stress and clinical supervision in mental health care. *Nursing Times* **92**(10): 34–5.

Faugier, J. and Butterworth, T. 1994 *Clinical Supervision. A Position Paper*. Manchester: Manchester University.

Fowler, J. 1995 Nurses' perceptions of the elements of good supervision. *Nursing Times* **91**(22): 33–7.

Handy, C. 1994 *The Empty Raincoat*. London: Hutchinson.

Hart, G.M. 1982 *The Process of Clinical Evaluation*. Baltimore, MD: University Press.

Hawkins, P. and Shohet, R. 1992 *Supervision in the Helping Professions*. Milton Keynes: Open University Press.

Johns, C. 1995 The value of reflective practice for nursing. *Journal of Clinical Nursing* **2**: 307–12.

Kohner, N. 1994 *Clinical Supervision in Practice*. London: King's Fund Centre.

Marinker, M. 1994 *Controversies in Health Care Policies*. London: BMJ Publishing.

NHSE (NHS Executive) 1992 *A Working Document; Revitalising the Strategy for Nursing*. London: NHSE.

Nicklin, P. 1997 Clinical supervision – Efficient and Effective? Unpublished conference paper, Jyvaskyla, Finland.

Norman, S. 1997 *Nursing Times Research,* **2**(2): 86–7 (Guest editorial).

Oojen, E.G. van 1996 Evidence Based Practice through Clinical Supervision. Unpublished CRNA Conference Paper, Oxford.

Paunonen, N. 1991 Changes initiated by a nursing supervision programme. *Journal of Advanced Nursing* **16**: 982–6.

Platt-Koch, L.M. 1986 Clinical supervision for psychiatric nurses. *Journal of Psychological Nursing* **26**(1): 7–15.

Proctor, B. 1992. In: Hawkins. P. and Shohet, R. (eds) *Supervision in the Helping Professions*. Milton Keynes: Open University Press.

Rafferty, M. and Coleman, M. 1996 Educating nurses to undertake clinical supervision in practice. *Nursing Standard* **10**(45): 38–41.

Revans, R. W. 1976 *Action Learning in Hospitals*. McGraw-Hill.

UKCC (United Kingdom Central Council for Nursing, Midwifery and Health Visiting) 1992 *Code of Conduct for the Nurse, Midwife and Health Visitor*. London: UKCC.

UKCC (United Kingdom Central Council for Nursing, Midwifery and Health Visiting) 1995 *Standards for Post-Registration Education and Practice* (PREP). London: UKCC.

UKCC (United Kingdom Central Council for Nursing, Midwifery and Health Visiting) 1996 *Position Statement on Clinical Supervision for Nursing and Health Visiting*. London: UKCC.

2

What Is Going On? Results of a Questionnaire

Veronica Bishop

In this chapter, data are presented which have been obtained from a questionnaire sent to all Trust Nurse Executives in England and Scotland, except for the 23 sites in the DoH-funded evaluation study carried out by Manchester University. While the data indicate a great deal of enthusiasm for clinical supervision, some concern must be shown by the lack of preparation and support for those involved in its implementation, a fact which will undoubtedly reflect badly in any useful evaluation exercise.

Introduction

One of the main reasons for producing this book is that I am constantly being asked by nurse managers and practitioners such questions as 'What is going on in clinical supervision?', 'How are people getting going with it?', 'Where do we start?' The lead from the DoH had been deliberately non-prescriptive, and the UKCC, quite properly in my view, maintained this stance. There is not, as yet, a recipe for success, and it would be wrong to expect different specialties and differently resourced localities to follow the same route. However, there is clearly a need to throw some thoughts into the common pool of ideas, and it is always helpful to consider where others are in any development and to learn of their successes and difficulties. This is particularly important at a time when the spirit of professional sharing is not encouraged by the internal market system. As professionals, we do not have the time, the money or the wish to repeat others' mistakes or to hold back progress by being overcautious. I knew, through my association with various Trusts and universities, that many in the nursing profession are ready to consider formalising the best of their practices, and clinical supervision offers a framework for this. Essentially, I wanted to know where clinical supervision was occurring, in the acute sector and in the community, and which specialties were involved. I also hoped to gain an insight into individual Trusts' commitment to clinical supervision and to identify how it was being managed in terms of time, funding and educational support.

Method

Through the auspices of Macmillan, the publishers, and the *Nursing Times Research* offices, I mailed a questionnaire to every named Trust Nurse Executive in England and Scotland, except for the 23 sites involved in the DoH-funded study (Butterworth *et al.*, 1997). The exclusion of Northern Ireland and Wales was not political in any way but merely a method of keeping the sample in line with other work and of accepting resource restrictions.

Knowing how busy Trust Nurse Executives are, and how much paper they have to deal with in a day, I designed the questionnaire on very simplistic lines. I was not hoping to obtain fine statistical data but rather 'outlines of activity', and, in view of this, the data should not be attributed any greater weight than is appropriate. A separate sheet was included for those who were not as yet, or did not intend to be, involved in clinical supervision. Free space was included for additional comments, and, to my delight, many people used this opportunity as well as offering contact names and telephone numbers for further discussion. Many questionnaires were filled in by the Trust Nurse Executives themselves, others had been passed to the named person responsible for taking clinical supervision forward and still others had been handed to non-designated personnel to fill in; generally the latter were the most incomplete. It must be said that, for a postal questionnaire with no reminders of any kind, the response rate was enviable, and I take this opportunity to thank everyone who responded.

Analysis

Of the 410 questionnaires sent out, I received 273 responses, giving a response rate of 67 per cent, which clearly indicated a strong interest in the subject and a commitment to contributing to the professional debate.

The questionnaire listed all the mainstream specialties, against which the respondent was to indicate which had clinical supervision implemented. Respondents added to these where applicable, showing a tremendous breadth of expertise reflecting not only traditional subdivisions of the nursing and health visiting professions, but also changing demands in the delivery of health care services and, significantly, the profession's diverse and innovative approaches to meeting those demands. Two groups undoubtedly under-represented are occupational health nurses and practice nurses, owing to the fact that they are not generally employed by Trusts. By the same token, nurses in many specialties within the independent sector will not have had the opportunity to give their views, which, given the size of that growing professional population, is regrettable and should be considered by policy-makers.

For convenience, in view of the varied allocation of specialties within Trusts, specialties were analysed under the broad headings:

- community Trusts;
- acute Trusts;
- mixed acute and community Trusts;
- very 'new' (under 6 months) clinical supervision sites;
- clinical supervision not implemented.

Figure 2.1 illustrates these groups as percentages of the overall response rate of the groups analysed.

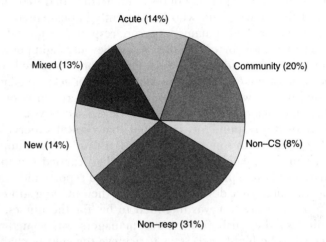

Acute (14%)

Mixed (13%)

Community (20%)

New (14%)

Non–CS (8%)

Non–resp (31%)

Non-CS, non-clinical supervision; Non-resp, non-respondent.

Figure 2.1 Response to questionnaire

Implementation of clinical supervision

Respondents indicated that some informal and formal mechanisms forming part of the processes of clinical supervision had been in operation for years in some clinical areas. The length of time over which clinical supervision was perceived to be practised in one way or another ranged from 11 years to 1 month, with a mean of 2.5 years in the community and 9 months in the acute sector. It is no surprise that the responses from the 'mixed' Trusts showed a mean between the other two groups of 1.8 years. It is reasonable to presume that our mental health colleagues have led the way here, and this is reflected in the community Trust replies and the involvement of community psychiatric nurses in clinical supervision.

Number of staff and lead person

The numbers of staff involved varied from 4000 to groups of five or six, the smaller numbers being more evident in the acute sector. Over 80 per cent of respondents in both the community and the (new) group who had recently implemented clinical supervision had a named person responsible for taking clinical supervision forward in their Trust. Seventy-eight per cent of the acute Trusts identified a named person, compared with 71 per cent of mixed Trusts. Questionnaires not acknowledging a named person were often incomplete and offered brief or no further information other than ticked or crossed boxes.

Many of the respondents indicated that clinical supervision had been piloted in some areas of the Trust rather than implemented in a blanket fashion, and some had carried out local evaluations of these pilots and kindly supplied reports and other supporting literature developed as part of their nursing strategy. While in most areas it was intended to be 'for the nurses, by the nurses', the push from nurse managers was sometimes perceived to be highly necessary to achieve the culture change required for effective peer review and support.

Supervisors

Four questions referred directly to supervisors, one of which was ambiguous, and many respondents went to great lengths to clarify their responses to the questions. Eighty-nine per cent of the mixed Trusts indicated that they gave their supervisors some training, ranging from in-house to outside, university-based support. Only slightly lower figures were suggested by the community and acute Trusts, but the 'new' group indicated that only 56 per cent of the supervisors were receiving any training.

The methods of selection of supervisors were very variable: some were self-selected, others were identified by management, and in some instances the supervisees selected them, with agreement from management. In some localities, a directory had been collated of suitable and willing supervisors, an innovation found to work well and one recommended in order to manage skill-sharing equably. Some supervision was given in groups, but data suggest that, more generally, it was given on a one-to-one basis, some supervisors meeting as many as nine individual supervisees. The mean figure, however, is less daunting, at six per supervisor. Sadly though, the figures for support for the supervisors do not reflect the concept that clinical supervision is for an entire professional life, as is demonstrated in Figure 2.2. However, where support systems for supervisors are in place, they have been well thought out and often linked both to an informal internal peer support system, and, more formally, to higher education.

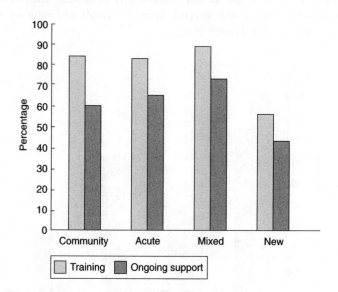

Figure 2.2   Supervisors: training and support

Supervisees

Over 85 per cent of responses obtained from the community and acute Trusts indicate that supervisees welcomed clinical supervision; however, only 69 per cent of the mixed Trusts gave a positive response to this question, and too few of the new sites answered to provide a meaningful figure. This same caution of the new sites was reflected in their responses to the question on the perceived benefits of clinical supervision, which is entirely proper given that most of them had implemented clinical supervision only within the past 3 months. The two cost-centred questions in this section referred to supervision being given during work time and whether that time was protected in the work agenda. Of the three established groups, 91 per cent of the community Trusts intended that clinical supervision should be carried out in work time, as did 90 per cent of the mixed Trusts and 85 per cent acute sector Trusts. However, the difference between intent and reality differed, 75 per cent of Trusts in the community achieving this, falling to 63 per cent in the mixed Trusts and 40 per cent in the acute sector (see Figure 2.3).

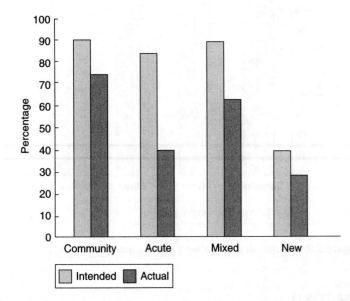

Figure 2.3   Supervisees: clinical supervision at work/time protected

Management

Over 90 per cent of the respondents in the community, acute and mixed groups intended to evaluate the effectiveness of clinical supervision, and similar figures were given in relation to the intent to keep clinical supervision on the agenda. However, only a little over half of the responses to the question on business planning indicated that clinical supervision was written into the corporate agenda or business plans of the Trust, even though many had it stated in clinical directorate strategies. Resources had rarely been identified, although pump-priming monies, educational funding, staff initiative resources and other *ad hoc* budgets were being used in some localities to train supervisors, run workshops and break new ground. Staff shortages were cited as a reason for blocking plans to implement clinical supervision and for increased workloads, particularly since the reduction of junior doctors' hours. The most common depressing feature about implementation of clinical supervision was the lack of funds to support what was perceived to be an important issue in nursing, particularly in the light of extended roles and staff shortages. Many additional comments referred to the acceptance of the concept and principles of clinical supervision by management but noted the lack of any concrete support to ensure its success, a deficiency commented on in relation to purchasing and contracting issues.

Problems in setting up clinical supervision

Time

The question 'What has been the biggest problem in setting up clinical supervision?' was answered by every respondent who had clinical supervision up if not entirely running. The most common reason given for difficulties was time: time constraints owing to workload, to staff shortages, to increased activity in contracts. One respondent added that, while the local purchasers in principle supported clinical supervision, they also had an agenda for increasing activity, and the two were not seen as necessarily compatible. One Trust experienced the opposite. The cost of the time anticipated to be taken up by clinical supervision had been calculated and funding allocated to employ staff to compensate for the lost activity. Sadly, poor recruitment meant that implementation still had not taken place.

Staff perceptions

A second, largely shared difficulty is that of clinical and managerial staff perceptions. Many facilitators found that staff were
unsure of what clinical supervision is and what is required to
achieve it. It is generally considered that the term 'supervision'
does nothing to reduce this confusion. Managers were often
unsure of how it 'fitted' with service priorities and questioned
the time and cost needed to implement it. Separating clinical
supervision from IPR and normal management functions
involved a great deal of time and effort from many respondents. As one respondent wrote:

> This trust has worked hard to ensure that clinical supervision is
> something done by nurses and is for nurses... I have personally
> spent a lot of time selling the idea that clinical supervision is not
> a management tool and is part and parcel of much of what is, [or
> should be], the normal role and function of the qualified nurse.

Another wrote:

> it is particularly difficult for... nurses to share their practice. Many
> skills are low visibility and afforded low status, and nurses have
> difficulty describing and analysing what they do. A lack of commonly
> accepted professional language and a lack of confidence are issues
> which need to be tackled both in the training of supervisors and in
> preparing practitioners to get the best out of clinical supervision.

Which model?

Selecting an achievable and workable model of supervision has
also presented many difficulties. The national lead was never
prescriptive, although some wished it had been, and the
suggested model based on the work of Proctor (1991), described
in the evaluation study at Manchester University, was not always
seen as helpful. Some saw it as too academic – was it the latest
academically driven 'buzz'? Others complained that it was too
vague. There was also some resistance to change, in the form
of 'We're doing it already', and one respondent went to some
length to explain this:

> There is confusion for those who have traditionally had time for
> reflection and peer review – what was new? How does this fit with

mentorship, preceptorship, appraisal and personal development and the host of other activities that can claim to be clinical supervision?

In admitting that these particular responses seemed cynical, the respondent went on to reflect that empowering nurses to achieve the best for patients was what any system must be about and that, if clinical supervision could pull all these concepts together, emphasising nurses' responsibility for PREP (UKCC, 1990) and *The Scope of Professional Practice* (UKCC, 1992), it was worth exploring. This view was certainly taken forward in one Trust, the respondent writing that he was particularly impressed at how nurses in specialist areas of care (diabetic, rheumatology, palliative care and breast care nurses, for example) had found clinical supervision helpful and had actively sought out their own clinical supervisors within their Trust.

Training for supervisees and supervisors

Many respondents identified the main difficulty with any model as being the preparation of staff and the need to consider some training for supervisees as well as supervisors, in order that maximum understanding and benefit could be gained from the system. The hierarchical nature of nursing presents difficulties in breaking down barriers in the selection of supervisors, and a shortage of suitable supervisors was raised in many of the responses. However, whether this was due to a lack of willingness of suitable staff, or to a lack of expertise, was not expressed, a point to which I shall return in the Discussion. Several respondents raised the more positive issue of a difficulty in meeting the demand for clinical supervision, particularly with respect to identifying sufficient supervisors without overloading individuals. Maintaining the momentum is seen as another common problem in steering the culture change necessary for clinical supervision to become integral to all practising nurses' agendas.

Private space

A trivial-sounding but important further difficulty common to many respondents is the lack of suitable venues for clinical supervision. Demands on space, even cupboards, for office or work use has stripped many localities bare of space for quiet, uninterrupted discourse. The removal of educational facilities is seen as one reason for this. Finding a space for two people to talk quietly seems a small matter, but such are the demands on space that some staff needs are not always accommodated.

The *key problems* identified by the questionnaire in the implementation of clinical supervision are:

- an ever-increasing workload;
- money for staff time and staff training;
- management and staff perceptions;
- training options and facilities for supervisors.

Perceived benefits of clinical supervision

The question 'What in your opinion is the main benefit of clinical supervision to your Trust?' was answered almost unanimously along similar lines by all groups who had implemented clinical supervision, whether the respondents were just starting or were well established in their strategy. Responses such as 'Enabling people to take action and believe that they can make a difference to practice' and 'ownership by the field staff has generated enormous enthusiasm, ideas and a strong reflective practice element' are common. Networking opportunities, and the development of a real body of professional expertise across boundaries and disciplines, are reported, and while it could be argued that these opportunities have always existed, clinical supervision has brought them into focus and made clinical supervision legitimate practice.

Recognition is given to the fact that increased activity often results in increased pressure, with the knock-on effect of threatening standards of care. Clinical supervision is acknowledged by many respondents as a method of ensuring that nursing practice is developed in conjunction with current thinking and agreed standards. Its value as a 'de-stressor' is emphasised, and some respondents regard it as an essential mechanism in risk management.

One Director of Nursing provided fuller comments than other respondents by stating that clinical supervision at her Trust is a culmination following on from clinical grading, skill-mixing and management reorganisation. This respondent had reduced the nursing management structure, some of the savings being used for clinical supervision posts which, in her view, resulted in improved professional support provided by credible role model practitioners. This is seen to have increased the confidence of staff and improved patient care. Valuing clinical practice is seen by many respondents as a major outcome of clinical supervision. Some considered that academic achievement had dominated our value system and welcomed the focus on care delivery and those providing it. Nonetheless, educational support for supervisors is an oft-stated requirement, and assistance from educational establishments in setting up awareness workshops, NVQs and degree pathways is seen as invaluable.

While it is not surprising that a self-selected population responded very enthusiastically about their progress – from those who were just starting out, to those who have travelled this road for a while – the validity of this response is to be seen in the high percentage of respondents. The real inroads have been made where staff who are committed to the principles of clinical supervision and optimistic of its value have formed focus groups and have created an impetus to drive the programme forward. Community respondents appear to be more confident in taking on the role of supervisor than do their acute sector colleagues, perhaps reflecting the autonomy that has long been part and parcel of many community staff. It may also be a reflection of the diversity of personal interactions required in community-based settings.

The key perceived improvements identified by respondents are those of enhanced patient care through clinical staff feeling supported and motivated, the raising of clinical aspects of health care that have previously been 'squeezed out' through management focus, and the promotion of informed clinical debate with both peers and other disciplines; of particular importance here is the identification of risk management and standard-setting.

The *key benefits*, perceived or evaluated, were:

- reflection on practice/staff confidence;
- support and valuing staff;
- improved clinical practice/competence;

- enhanced service provision;
- personal and professional growth;
- happier staff/improved morale;
- a reduced risk to staff and patients;
- increased staff motivation/commitment;
- the potential to assist with staff recruitment and retention;
- a reduction in sickness rates;
- improved and increased communication;
- reduced stress levels.

Those not currently involved in clinical supervision

This minority group of respondents is not sleeping! Of the 30 respondents, all but one were intending to review their stance on clinical supervision. The few exceptions already had several mechanisms, such as mentorship, preceptorship and IPR, in place and did not see the need to modify or add to this programme. One respondent identified a clinical occupational psychologist as a staff support resource; another was committed to Investors in People and IPR. Some of the respondents had just begun to pilot clinical supervision and would have been justified in filling in the main questionnaire, while others were debating the issue within their nursing strategies. Particular concerns raised by this group reflect those already participating in clinical supervision – these are issues of time and resources, particularly where nursing establishments have been cut and the skill-mix tightened.

Discussion

Getting going

The high response rate to the questionnaire indicates a profound interest across the health care services in clinical supervision. While some Trusts were awaiting the results of the DoH-funded Manchester evaluation study before committing themselves to implementing clinical supervision, others had bitten the bullet and got on with it, convinced that some mech-

anism had to be pulled together to support nurses through
the many challenges and changes currently (and for the foreseeable future) impacting on the profession. There has been
some reluctance or difficulty in introducing clinical supervision, particularly in general nursing settings, as most of the
current literature stems from mental health settings and is not
easily transferred to other settings. Heather Davies, while at
the Welsh Office as a Clinical Effectiveness Advisor, explained
this further in a personal communication (1979):

> Mental health settings are focused largely around the therapeutic
> relationship between the patient and the nurse, therefore clinical
> supervision should largely focus on what the nurse brings to that
> relationship. However, to achieve 'healing' in general nursing the
> nurse is required to develop a nurse/patient relationship that allows
> for identification of problems from which interventions can be
> determined. This high level of factual knowledge and skill requires
> a supervisor who has both insight into the interpersonal dynamic
> process and can also, through the reflective process, enable the nurse
> to identify knowledge and skill deficits.

The issue of injecting enthusiasm for clinical supervision and
having, to some degree, achieved it, and then to sustain and
develop this cultural change, is a frequent concern of respondents. Some identified that a core of committed staff is essential to move implementation programmes forward and share
across localities the issues that arise. Such a group needs access
to those who are well versed in the theory and practice of clinical supervision as a resource.

Comments unremittingly highlight the two sides of the clinical supervision coin: its value to patient care through an
empowered and supported clinical staff, and its cost in terms
of staff time. The latter would, some respondents indicated,
be considerably eased if a robust costing mechanism could be
identified that could be set against hard outcomes, thus offering
currency at the purchasing counter. However, the view voiced
by one respondent was that formalising peer review had cut
down on many *ad hoc* meetings and thus effected a saving in
resources. Other respondents, while not ignoring the cost implications, considered that clinical supervision was essential to
sound practice and the development and maintenance of standards and patient safety, particularly in high-activity areas.

Could one afford not to implement it, particularly in the context of evidence-based practice, audit and risk management? The point was raised that clinical supervision had been going on informally in some areas of mental health, uncosted but totally as the norm.

Many respondents, in particular the smaller Trusts, have adopted the 'softly, softly' approach, which allows for a gradual change in attitudes of clinical staff and managers, and causes minimal initial effect on finances by implementing clinical supervision in selected areas. It also facilitates some evaluative component within the overall trust or directorate strategy of a manageably sized group. Several respondents attached profiles of their Trust programme for clinical supervision and its evaluation. The high commitment to evaluation in itself would be heartening were it not for the fact that, particularly in the acute sector, there is some resistance to protecting the time allocated to clinical supervision. There are inferences in the responses that supervisees often feel guilty at taking the 'time out', and I have certainly received plenty of anecdotal evidence to support this.

For those still on the brink of setting out protocols for clinical supervision, it would seem to be good advice to settle for less but ensure that it is upheld.

In other words, if 1 hour per month seems to pose insurmountable difficulties in terms of resources, aim for 1 hour every 2 months. Only by ensuring that clinical supervision is embedded in the system, and not waived aside, can staff be properly supported in their work and the effectiveness of clinical supervision be evaluated. Consider the results of the questionnaire – almost everyone is going to evaluate clinical supervision but few have secured one of the essential components for its effectiveness, that of time.

Identifying supervisors

A lack of suitable people as a resource for supervisors is a common finding in the responses, and I found myself wondering whether we are undervaluing ourselves – thus maintaining the habit of a lifetime! In considering the requirements of an effective clinical supervisor, we must leave our hierarchical baggage behind and look to offer all registered practitioners the opportunity to develop their supervisory skills. The generally agreed target for supervisors is that of a safe, competent and experienced qualified nurse with good listening skills and the ability to give constructive feedback, as well as a willingness to assume the role and responsibilities of a clinical supervisor. One Trust, developing clinical supervision in conjunction with its local university, stated specific criteria for supervisors, these being willingness and aptitude, as well as the necessity for supervisors to be qualified for at least 3 years and have 1 year's experience in their specialty. Identifying supervisors for some senior nurses and in some specialties, especially in rural areas, must present particular problems, but some respondents have used their networking skills and are involving nurses and members of other disciplines. This multidisciplinary approach to clinical supervision, where adopted, is seen to have a highly beneficial effect not only on team working, but also in broadening discussions. Some models of clinical supervision being used include those of radiologists, speech therapists and occupational therapists, and in these cases this cross-disciplinary dimension is seen as very beneficial. One respondent wrote:

> we realised at an early stage that we needed to develop a sound knowledge base for all trained practitioners... and have provided training at various levels from a one day 'awareness' to a degree level module... our progress is slow but generally consistent.

She went on to say that there is a need to sustain the momentum and provide a variety of resources which should, ideally, be headed by a facilitator.

Contracting and setting standards

Some respondents stressed the need for confidentiality of information exchanged at clinical supervision sessions and described a written contracting procedure between supervisors and supervisees to ensure that all parties involved were clear on the ground rules.

Several respondents stated that they had a standard for clinical supervision that applied to both qualified and unqualified staff. Some localities have incorporated clinical supervision as a formal part of staff job descriptions, thus putting a managerial commitment to the concept strongly in place. Many respondents see themselves, quite rightly, as pioneers in the field of clinical supervision. The concept has been strongly promoted nationally, and suggestions have been made on how to set about it, but the real challenge for any clinical area is to cut the principles and goals into a shape that fits their resources and expertise without losing the overall thrust and benefit to be gained. What comes across strongly from the respondents is an enormous commitment to a pragmatic approach in applying the concept of clinical supervision to practice. The need for clinical supervision appears to be undisputed, although the terminology may be.

Conclusion

The respondents to my questionnaire are pioneers. They have taken the opportunity and moved nursing forward, by pushing and dragging, towards the real culture of a profession – critique, excellence and recognition. In order not to lose this powerhouse, we must identify the best in what is being tried – and here the Butterworth study (Butterworth *et al.*, 1997) is invaluable as the measurements taken from across 23 sites derive from the same instruments – but it must be remembered that such a study was a complete innovation in its time and, as such, is limited in its findings: it cannot be expected to answer all the questions being asked. Given the acceptance of the need for clinical supervision, and acknowledging the tremendous work that has flowed from this recognition, what can we do not to lose all the developing expertise, not to let clinical supervision become another 'nursing process', a flavour of the year?

The answer lies, I suspect, in the core values that every respondent to the questionnaire indicated that they held dear: valuing staff, improving staff and striving for excellence in care provision. These core values are achieved by support, education and standard-setting through a variety of mechanisms, including clinical supervision. The success of this mechanism is, in very large part, dependent on the supervisor, and this is to a large degree recognised by respondents. What is less clear is the identification of the skills required for good supervision and the involvement of counselling, monitoring and challenge. And what preparation should be given to nurses to do this? How would you know if someone employed from another Trust had supervisory skills that were in line with yours? This takes us to the serious issue of supporting supervisors. We cannot find ourselves in the position of expecting a group of people to carry the burden of the profession's anxieties and learning processes unaided – that is setting us all up for failure.

References

Butterworth, T., Carson, J., White, E., Jeacock, J., Clements, A. and Bishop, V. 1997 *It Is Good to Talk. An Evaluation of Clinical Supervision and Mentorship in England and Scotland.* Manchester: University of Manchester School of Nursing and Midwifery.

Hawkins, P. and Shohet , R. 1992 *Supervision in the Helping Professions.* Milton Keynes: Open University Press.

Proctor, B. 1991 On being a trainer and supervision for counselling in action. In: Dryden, W. and Thorne, B. *Training and Supervision for Counselling in Action.* London: Sage.

UKCC (United Kingdom Central Council for Nursing, Midwifery & Health Visiting) 1990 *The Report of the Post-Registration Education and Practice Project (PREPP).* London: UKCC.

UKCC (United Kingdom Central Council for Nursing, Midwifery & Health Visiting) 1992 *The Scope of Professional Practice.* London: UKCC.

3

Introducing Clinical Supervision and Beginning Evaluation

Chris Maggs

Tell me I am doing it right, just doing it well, sometimes, please.

There is widespread interest in the development and implementation of clinical supervision. The movement appears to have been led from the 'top', which may have caused some anxieties at clinical level as practitioners seek to take clinical supervision on board. This paper traces the piloting of three approaches to clinical supervision and reviews the process through which nurses in one acute Trust explored their practice and clinical supervision. The method chosen was the 'master class' approach, using an external expert. The paper provides practical help in bringing about change and also reflects on the 'politics' of clinical supervision for the nursing profession.

Introduction

Clinical supervision, in whatever form, is with the profession for the foreseeable future. It would appear to offer, as a minimum, an opportunity to reorientate professional relationships away from the conventional hierarchical model and towards the collegial or, more impressively, partnership model for practice. Considerable anxieties have been unleashed by its promulgation, not least about its operation in practice and its relationship to managerialism. As always, there have been questions raised about how 'it' will be paid for and whether 'we' can afford it. More importantly, there seems to be a political agenda – be this within the top echelons of the profession or, more probably, among its most vocal protagonists – that clinical supervision will be a reality, come what may. Yet, as with many changes in the profession of nursing in the UK, nurses and nursing manage to try to shoot the messenger and 'rubbish' the message.

Other contributors to this volume explore the conceptual and professional values and frameworks of clinical supervision; this chapter records the experiences of nurses in one provincial general hospital NHS Trust as they were introduced to and came to understand clinical supervision and its relevance to their professional lives. Before exploring this, it might be useful to set out the stance taken by this contributor to clinical supervision.

It would appear to be a commonplace that change in nursing in the UK is invariably driven by groups with access to professional power but without an overall ideological or theoretical perspective. This style of 'leadership' depends on individuals with considerable communication skills and access to communication networks but, more importantly, access to key players at the centre of professional power. This may not be a 'bad' thing, and the fact that the rank and file have to be educated or persuaded is the familiar lot of the 'radical' or revolutionary. There is, however, an alternative. As liberation theology shows and critical theory illuminates, actions that derive from the experience of the social group – in this case nurses – are not merely unpredictable but subversive, creative and uncontrollable.

Clinical supervision, no matter what the intentions of those who first explored its usefulness to nursing, has become, or is about to become, another instance of professional repression. Debates about how it should be modelled, whether it should be based on existing clinical grade hierarchies, whether to engage in clinical supervision as a supervisor or supervisee, and what training and support, if any, are needed are all, to this author's mind, indicators of attempts to control what might well be a liberating moment.

To take personal responsibility within a collective ideology for patient care is what being a nurse is about, but unless there is an exposition of that ideology (or, as our teachers would have it, a theory) of nursing, such endeavours have the hallmarks of competence rather than capability.

As a first step, it is necessary for nurses themselves to begin to express their thoughts about the circumstances: their relationships with patients, with each other and especially with those who 'supervise' their practice. We could argue whether that expression can arise spontaneously or needs some individual 'facilitator' or event to trigger it, but the issues remain the same. There needs to be such an expression, and it cannot be imposed.

Thereafter, what happens becomes uncertain unless someone or something intervenes to control events. We can either be part of that unfolding drama or be part of the controlling mechanism; what we cannot do is to walk away, for that is also part of the process of control.

With these thoughts in mind, nurses at one provincial acute hospital Trust came together to debate clinical supervision and the way forward – or rather, they came together to debate many things while attending a series of meetings about clinical supervision. We shall return to this difference of the view of events later.

The hospital

The Trust employs about 1300 nurses (full and part time) and consists of a large site in a county town together with a small community hospital some 7 miles away. Nurses tend to work at one or other site and see each other only at formal gatherings, for example senior nurse conferences. The hospital has a centralised nursing budget and an embryonic form of clinical directorates. It, like many Trusts, experiences financial pressures to reduce costs and seek cost improvement programmes, currently having a substantial deficit despite attempts to 'do things smarter'.

The Executive Nurse and Chief Executive have a history of support for the profession and for finding creative and innovative ways to develop practice. There has been a research and development (R&D) department for more than 5 years, members of which are engaged in clinical research and development projects both within and outside the hospital. The Trust has made a number of joint appointments with the local university School of Health to support R&D, education and training.

Late in 1995, the R&D department, as part of its agenda for 1995/96, agreed to lead discussion in the hospital about clinical supervision. The way in which it decided to do this was by inviting an external moderator to chair a series of 'master classes' with representatives of nurses working in the hospital. The master classes were also to include one to which senior nurse managers were invited. The next section describes what happened.

The rationale for the master class approach

The master class approach was deliberately chosen to provide an opportunity for the nurses in this Trust to work their way through many of the stages that others, especially those at policy level in the profession, had travelled in their journey towards clinical supervision. This was particularly important for the exploration of what constituted clinical practice, professional accountability and autonomy of practice.

The master class approach exposes individuals or small groups to debate with an acknowledged expert who, through challenge and support, moves the participants to a new and higher understanding of their role while retaining the unique contribution and perspective that the individual brings to practice. In this case, the moderator is an acknowledged expert in clinical supervision with a wealth of experience of similar debates and discussion at the clinical level within the nursing profession, as well as a deep understanding of the policy agendas.

Participants have to recognise that expert as an expert, and, in this case, the evidence for that expertise could not be first hand. Expertness was demonstrated by the moderator's biography and introduction to the participants. Key examples of 'expertness' were identified in the introduction, and participants were encouraged to challenge the moderator's credentials. While some may have had private reservations or questions about that degree of expertise, none was voiced in the sessions.

The master class approach requires participants first to show where they currently are in their roles and skills and then, challenged by the moderator, to respond and revise these upwards. This can be fairly 'global', for example in a philosophy of care, or fairly discrete, for example record-keeping and accountability. Master classes move between levels while keeping the overarching goal – in this case nursing practice – constantly in mind. The expectation is that progress will be made towards that goal, but it is also acknowledged that the process is a learning activity and that participants will achieve different outcomes and levels of insight.

Three separate half-day sessions were set aside and, by means of a personal letter to each nurse in the hospital, nurses were invited to choose the most suitable event to attend. In the event, the three groups were about the same size (approximately 45–50 nurses each), the groups reflecting the grading profile of the nursing establishment. The sessions were held in the afternoon, generally agreed to be easier for nurses to attend, in the newly opened nurses' lecture theatre in the postgraduate medical centre.

The letter of invitation briefly introduced the notion of clinical supervision and set out the format for the discussions. Other than that, no preliminary work was done with those attending or their colleagues in the clinical areas.

Each session was addressed by the external moderator, an acknowledged expert in developing clinical supervision who had been responsible for developing the DoH's view on clinical supervision and was involved in a study of the implementation of clinical supervision in England.

We are all familiar with attending or organising workshops and have experience of the importance of planning for the event and of the problems that can arise. In this case, it was agreed that the moderator would want to encourage as much participation as possible from those attending, since this was the purpose of the event. Too large an audience would inhibit discussion, one too small might feel threatening to some. Breaking up larger audiences into small groups is a common approach to encouraging discussion but can limit the interaction being sought, and so-called 'plenary sessions' often fall flat as each group tries to 'report back' on its discussions.

As always, compromises need to be made. We adopted the format of the large, initial group then breaking into smaller groups. The discussions in the large group ranged far and wide, which was encouraged by the moderator; the small groups were asked, however, to focus specifically on clinical supervision, but even then the groups' conversations covered much contextual ground.

The introduction by the moderator to the whole group rehearsed the recent history of clinical supervision and the national picture of its introduction, outlining some of the key issues surrounding the concept and its implementation. The moderator took pains not to present any formed views of how clinical supervision might be constituted, whether it was desirable or not, or how it might be taken forward.

The discussions were rather more wide ranging than might have been expected. Nurse after nurse spoke of the current problems of delivering best practice, the pressures to 'cut corners', the anxieties of not doing the best for patients, the guilt at not being able really to care for patients as they wished.

Many of these themes and comments will be familiar and find expression wherever and whenever nurses have an opportunity for discussion. However, the groups had come together specifically to discuss clinical supervision and, in smaller groups, they began to explore what clinical supervision might mean to them. The small groups were self-selecting, although most seemed to be made up not of friends or work colleagues, but of relatively random grouping of those present. This helped, to some extent, to make sure that these smaller groups continued to have an opportunity to challenge each other without splitting along clinical area or arbitrary grading lines.

Discussions in the master classes

Before looking in some detail at the views expressed in the master classes, it is worthwhile making two preliminary remarks. First, in her report on clinical supervision in five NDUs, Kohner (1994) makes a series of comments about nurses' attitudes to the idea of clinical supervision, which were, unknowingly, repeated by nurses at the master classes. The following section sets out those thoughts, and the reader will be able to make the connection between events at the Trust and those described by Kohner. Second, no-one present at the master classes could recall a recent instance of receiving a compliment on their work by a colleague of any level of seniority, nor, perhaps more importantly given that they recognised the need (because they raised it themselves unprompted) had any one given any compliments to another, except in a very vague way of unspecified courtesy at 'handover' time. Both examples point to and reinforce the need expressed by Kohner and others for a substantial and more general cultural change to accompany and sustain clinical supervision in practice.

That view can be substantiated, in part, by the way in which the master classes proceeded. The rationale for the master classes has already been discussed above; here it is useful to note that participants were often slow to contribute to the discussions in open sessions and found small group work more congenial. While there may be good reasons for suggesting that was inevitable – small groups ought to work better – it is also the case that the participants found the events quite challenging and daunting. Many came to the events, it seemed, to be 'told what to do, what was going on', and this appears to be common when nurses meet in such numbers. The management style and professional culture are part of the reason for these expectations. When confronted by a master class format that required them to examine their own and each other's practice, many turned inward and back to the formulaic approach of such sessions. Fortunately, one advantage of the master class style lies in the presence of the 'master", the expert who is knowledgeable not just about the topic, but also about the process of facilitation and learning. As time elapsed, whether in the small groups or in the plenary sessions, more and more participants became more and more vocal and assertive about their practice and its setting.

The nurses who attended came with a mix of views about what clinical supervision might be and how it might – or might not – work for them. For example, some thought it was similar to the supervision that midwives experienced; others that it was another form of management performance review. For some, the concept was vague and woolly, and they wanted the moderator to tell them what it was and how it would work in practice. Still others felt that they wanted to explore a wider agenda about professional accountability and professional autonomy before getting to grips with what they saw, with suspicion, as another 'fad' or fashion.

Clinical supervision was seen by participants as offering 'something', in particular 'something for them'. That something was elusive, and there was a general sense of suspicion about what it might be and whence the offer originated. At a crucial and early stage in the master class discussions, participants addressed the issue of 'Why?' They came up with a series of reasons for nurses, including closer links between practice and continuing professional education, increased morale among staff and a sense of sharing expertise. There was also the sense of relief that it would be 'all right' for nurses to take time out for themselves, 'to take time to think about me'. However, the most vocal part of that discussion came when debating the benefits to patients of clinical supervision.

Many participants argued that clinical supervision would help them to 'advance patient care into the future' through improved quality of care, evidence-based practice and better value for money from nursing practice. This would be supported by clinical supervision, which would give nurses the skills necessary for risk management and innovative practice. The cultural change brought about by a supportive but questioning climate would help staff to be more receptive to sharing and goal-setting. Importantly, participants spoke of the relationship between clinical supervision and clinical leadership, suggesting that the two were intertwined.

Participants identified obstacles to autonomous practice and professional accountability. These included the current system for nursing management, the lack of knowledge of key issues for the Trust and for the nursing agenda in the Trust, the lack of clarity about the national picture in nursing policy and a sense of local isolation.

It was pointed out that a system of clinical IPR already seemed to be designed to address some of the aspects of the perceived version of clinical supervision and that another system would introduce further stress and pressure on valuable clinical time. Worries were expressed about the commitment of the senior management to clinical supervision or, indeed, to any form of autonomous working practice. There was a strong sentiment that, even if the nurses grasped the nettle of clinical supervision, there would be little management support for them.

The latter became a particular issue and focus when participants discussed how it would work in practice. Participants generated a catalogue of activities that they saw as non-clinical but which had to be completed – for example audits for the health authority including the 'named nurse' audit – that did not appear to be directly geared to practice. How, participants asked, could they take on another activity within the existing establishment and within the existing time available for care? What estimates were there for the time that clinical supervision would demand if it were to be introduced correctly and used effectively to change monitor and practice?

Participants were also sceptical about the methods for clinical supervision. They had discussed a variety of ways in which it might be structured, for example a traditional hierarchical model and a peer review model, but they worried about confidentiality, what would happen if 'bad practice' was identified, who would need to know about the results of any supervision, and so on.

The more senior participants wanted to know the implications for skill mix and for resources within the clinical area. Increased throughput, shorter stays and increased patient dependency levels were pressures that had already stretched the nursing resource. Another demand without commensurate resources might be too much for the clinical areas to bear.

Some participants asked whether every nurse would be required to undergo clinical supervision or whether it was truly an option. Some felt that unless everyone participated, it would not have the desired effect, although the precise definition of that effect or its outcome was not easily identified by the groups. Others felt that it should be voluntary to the extent that individual nurses should be able to opt in or out and identify the model that best suited their practice and clinical area.

The issue of training as a supervisor, or indeed as a supervisee, was addressed, participants generally agreeing that the supervisor should receive training, not least because of the issues of confidentiality raised by clinical supervision. There was also the need to help supervisors deal with the need to 'counsel' supervisees, skills which many felt they lacked, at least in this context.

Participants at the master classes asked, 'Who will supervise the supervisors?' There was a general sense at the end of the sessions that a hierarchical model would be introduced and that the more senior nurses would, themselves, need to experience clinical supervision. However, the emphasis was on the clinical component, and, they asked, how would a line nurse manager clinically supervise a senior clinical nurse?

The close links between the local university School of Health and the Trust were acknowledged to be a source of strength in implementing clinical supervision in the Trust. Any educational activity needed to help its introduction could be accredited through the ENB Higher Award modular framework, and staff at the School were supportive of clinical supervision. Given that the Trust has an R&D department within the Nursing Directorate, participants expected considerable support and guidance from the R&D staff if they were to proceed. There was a sense in which experimentation should happen before any fixed model or models could be agreed; the R&D department had the expertise and experience to permit that experimentation to be properly evaluated.

Review of findings from the master classes

The discussion and the statements demonstrate this process of learning, described in the rationale for the master classes, in action. For example, the sessions started by asking participants about current practice, confidence in its effectiveness and approaches to professional accountability. The sessions also included, as part of the introduction and the development of confidence in the expert, a short overview of policy and clinical supervision, but this did not include any definitions, models or examples of preferred practice. Participants responded by unpacking many of the issues they faced in delivering good nursing care and some of the obstacles to and supportive structures in good practice.

The end result of the sessions was a general resolve to continue the discussion but in the clinical areas. Some felt ready to embark on the implementation of clinical supervision, and some decided it was not for them. Among the senior managers, the sense was to take matters slowly, to see what if any resources might be needed and where they might come from, to work with any clinical area that wanted to take matters forward, while continuing to support those who were either unsure or did not wish to participate.

All present agreed that clinical supervision was not an end in itself but one means for enabling good practice and professional accountability.

The next steps

A report was written by the moderator for the Executive Nurse and circulated to the clinical nursing staff and to the Dean and lecturers of the School of Health. The report recommended experimentation in seeking ways to monitor and support good clinical practice and the need for an evaluation of any initiatives undertaken by nurses in the Trust.

Within a week, three clinical areas had identified an interest in taking the initiative forward and expressed a willingness to be part of an evaluation framework. Each identified a different way of proceeding: one wanted to continue the existing clinical IPR system, another to have a hierarchical model of clinical supervision, and the third to have a collaborative and collegial model. They all sought help in developing their thoughts and working out how to evaluate their achievements.

Members of the R&D department who were already associated with these clinical areas liaised with them about clinical supervision. The predominant request was for further informal discussions about clinical supervision, particularly with nurses who had been unable to attend the master classes, followed by the need for training in supervision.

The nurses also wanted to explore ways in which they might record the process and outcomes of clinical supervision, particularly in light of their wish that both process and outcome should remain confidential. While they would continue to take part in clinical IPR (and indeed wished to incorporate it into clinical supervision and record-keeping), they felt that some other documentary record was necessary for clinical supervision.

There was also a general feeling that, once the decision to proceed had been made, some mechanism needed to be in place to assess the effects on clinical practice and on the individual's performance. How, they asked, could a baseline be established against which change could be measured?

The pilot study

It was agreed to establish a pilot study that would explore models of clinical supervision and ways of evaluating their effect on practice. The three areas agreed to participate, and a protocol was devised for the pilot project. The aim of the project was to improve practice, the objectives being to establish mechanisms for clinical supervision, to assess the impact of each model on clinical practice and to disseminate the findings to the Trust nurses.

Each clinical area set up its own group to take the matter forward with the support of a member of the R&D staff. Each devised a programme for the implementation of their approach and a timetable for action. Each group also explored how it might 'measure' the impact of clinical supervision or changes in practice as a result of the initiative. All agreed that measurement would be difficult, and the early results of a survey of the literature did not really identify a way forward. The advice from the R&D department staff was that 'evaluation' in the classical sense was extremely difficult to carry out in this case if nurses were after some sort of proof that clinical supervision 'worked'. In discussions with the link R&D person, the nurses in each area were advised to concentrate on stating their own objectives for clinical supervision simply and clearly, for example 'Each nurse will have a supervisor for clinical supervision allocated' or 'Each nurse will experience clinical supervision within a stated time period.'

It was agreed that, for the purposes of the clinical areas, a general statement of the standards of nursing care they believed they were achieving, together with a statement of their expectations, would suffice. These statements would be reviewed after 1 year of piloting. In addition, information about patient satisfaction audits, staff sickness and absence rates, clinical IPR and access and uptake of continuing education events could also be considered as possible indicators of change. The groups rejected any more formal measures such as stress rating scales as being either too complicated or not immediately relevant.

External evaluation is, arguably, more systematic and rigorous than internal review or evaluation. However, the external evaluation to be carried out by the R&D department as part of its programme of activity for the year also faced the same problems of methodology and suitable research instruments, as did the clinical staff. In addition, the external evaluation required the explicit statement of intent by the participants in order that it could be evaluated, and there was little to suppose that such a clear statement would be forthcoming or that it would not substantially alter in the light of experience.

The external evaluation, therefore, encompasses those issues raised by the pilot projects and uses the same indicators but, additionally, explores the Trust-wide perspective and how the development of clinical supervision meets the nursing agenda set by the Trust for the same period.

Preliminary results

The three models have previously been referred to, a little more detail will usefully be added here so that the early stages may be better understood.

The Trust established clinical IPR more than 3 years before it considered the issue of clinical supervision. Initially an annual appraisal linked to clinical skills and continuing education needs, the clinical IPR system has undergone considerable modification and sophistication since it was first introduced. An Assistant Director of Nursing Services attached to the R&D department has responsibility for ensuring that all nurses complete their clinical IPR each year; the format has been changed, and the ENB 10 key characteristics are used to provide a benchmark for assessment. Nurses personally identify their existing level of clinical competencies against the key characteristics, and this is agreed in discussion with the immediate line, clinical manager. Continuing education needs and clinical aspirations are identified, together with their rationale and a timescale for their achievement. This then forms the basis for clinical development for the coming year. In all of this, the nurse has in mind the annual nursing agenda and the aims of the particular clinical directorate in which he or she works. The most recent edition of the form questions the nurse about clinical supervision and asks for at least two examples of benefits to the nurse of the experience of clinical supervision. This, then, forms the basis of one model, the *status quo* model.

The second model adopted was the hierarchical model. In this case, each nurse was supervised by the immediate clinical superior, based on clinical grading. Thus, a staff nurse graded at E grade would be supervised by a nurse graded F. Wherever possible, the supervisor and supervisee would work similar shift patterns to ensure clinical contact and continuity.

The final model, the collegial model, involved all nurses meeting regularly, but not necessarily frequently, to discuss their own and each other's practice in a general discussion. This model implies time to meet as a group, and the clinical area that chose this approach felt that it was able to do so because of the shift patterns worked in the department.

Of the three groups or models, two are up and running, and the third, the collegial/collaborative model, is still under discussion. This probably reflects the complexity of the model, which may run counter to the way in which nursing is currently organised – hierarchically – and the need to develop confidence that a collaborative and supportive structure is possible.

All staff have completed the first round of clinical IPR since the start of the pilot (they had completed a similar exercise for the previous year), and a system of periodic audit of the indicators has been set in place.

Nurses in the two working models received, as requested, further information and then training in supervision, including the role of the supervisee, and the relevant member of the R&D staff continues to attend the meetings of the 'steering groups' for each model. To date, little is obviously happening, and there have been no problems encountered other than the perennial one of finding time in the working week for supervision.

Conclusion

Introducing clinical supervision is not a great challenge, as this pilot project shows. Many nurses are open to new ideas, especially if they offer a chance to improve standards of care and appear to offer new ways of working. The demand for further training, in this case for supervisor and supervisee roles, is a concomitant of change in the profession. Most are now well used to setting aims and objectives, creating a timescale for change and including mechanisms for evaluating developments. That much can be said to be the end result of many years of audit, standard-setting and quality initiatives, as well as the outcome of continuing professional education.

A number of reservations may be inserted at this point. First, there does not seem to be evidence of the nurse's ability to transfer knowledge and skills acquired in one setting to another. During the discussions about roles, a number of participants made the point that the new supervisor role would require skills in communication, honesty, openness, confidentiality, the ability to handle people, time management and many other areas of knowledge. Few argued that they already had these skills and could transfer them, with little further input, to the new situation. Instead, there was almost universal call for more training. It is easy to acknowledge but difficult to understand the emphasis on demands for training in this context, especially since the calls are for training associated with, for example, 'skills' to do with confidentiality. It might reasonably be assumed that all nurses are grounded in the need for confidentiality but, as in many other cases, the demands still are made for training.

Second, the pace of development is predictable, but only if the model chosen is 'off the shelf', as in the case of the two sites that are currently up and running at the Trust. This is in part because there is a literature that is accessible to newcomers, and the pitfalls and processes are usually well defined and explored. In the case of the third site, which is exploring a more challenging model that runs counter to the way in which nursing is traditionally organised and which calls for major strides in 'working together', the pace of change is slow, uneven and unpredictable. Both for the nurses involved and for their managers, this appears to be frustrating, especially when they see their colleagues forging ahead, and there is the possibility that they will decide to abandon their chosen path and follow a more well-trodden one. Such a decision would be consistent, in one sense, with choice and with autonomous practice. However, nursing theorists (in particular Rosemary Parse) and others (Habermass, 1971) have something to offer such nurses that may help them continue their chosen way.

Whatever the contrary appears in the rhetoric of clinical supervision, the fact remains that it will soon figure as part of the 'quality assurance' process for contracting for nursing care in the NHS. In the absence of other indicators of nursing effectiveness, commissioners and others will substitute issues such as clinical supervision into their audit of care. As with the 'named nurse', so too might clinical supervision become an exercise. This will be despite the feelings and knowledge of many in the profession that it should play a central role in their clinical life, that it does offer an opportunity to show personal and professional accountability for nursing care. It may well be that pressure to meet targets for the introduction of clinical supervision will lead to its development being led not by nurses but by employers. A consequence of that drift will be to seek the easier options, the models that can be introduced within given timescales and can be 'shown' to be in place.

The great adventure lies in the unknown, those places where control is stripped away and nurses as nurses and as people begin to set their own agendas for 'human becoming' (Parse, 1992). The third group in the Trust is confronting, wittingly or unwittingly, this greater challenge – to see the connections between clinical supervision and professional autonomy. The master classes provided the stimulus but none of the answers nor any real guidance. They are very much alone in the endeavour, even though they can call on support. They are beginning to explore their boundaries as people and as nurses, it is uncomfortable and uncertain, and the rewards are not clear. However, the potential for their practice and for the discipline of nursing in unimaginable.

Finally, we must recognise the words and sentiments expressed by so many of the nurses taking part in this 'experiment', not specifically about clinical supervision nor how it might work in practice, but about themselves. The chapter opened with a plea, spoken by one and echoed by many – 'Tell me I am doing it right, just doing it well, sometimes, please.' If we did, we might perhaps not need to embark on this course at all.

References

Habermass, J. 1971 *Knowledge of Human Interests*. Boston: Beacon Press.

Kohner, N. 1994 *Clinical Supervision in Practice*. London: King's Fund Centre

Parse, R.R. 1992 Human becoming: Parse's theory of nursing. *Nursing Science Quarterly*, **5**: 35–42.

4

Snapshots from Scotland

Jeannette Davidson

This chapter describes investment at national level in Scotland which has encouraged developments in reflective practice and nursing audit. This includes the Strategy for Nursing, Midwifery and Health Visiting in Scotland Project, the Scottish Nursing Audit Project and the distance learning programme *Moving to Audit: An Education Package for Nurses, Midwives and Health Visitors* (University of Dundee Centre for Medical Education, 1994). It questions what is understood by the term 'clinical supervision' and goes on to recount the thinking of the NHS Trust Directors of Nursing Services Group on clinical supervision. It then describes the different approaches to the implementation of clinical supervision adopted by one health board directly managed unit, two NHS trusts and one education provider. These descriptions are first-hand accounts provided specifically for this chapter by nurses involved in devising these approaches.

Introduction

Anyone considering recent developments in the nursing professions in Scotland for the first time might easily assume that clinical supervision arrived here by post in 1993. That was when *A Vision for the Future* (Department of Health, 1993), a document produced by the DoH NHSE in England, in consultation with English nurses and health visitors, English NHS Trust Chief Executives and the English National Board, was distributed to NHS Trust Directors of Nursing in Scotland.

This is because, as others have said, Scotland's relationship with England is like that of a man sharing a bed with an elephant (Scott, 1985): the elephant is likely to crush its bedfellow. This can happen quite by accident without evil intent just because of the sheer size of the elephant.

For this reason, the opportunity is taken at the start of this chapter to sketch out something of activities in Scotland that have contributed to the present position on clinical supervision.

Background

Strategy

What many believe to have been the most turbulent period in the evolution of the NHS began in 1988. It was then that the Chief Nursing Officer for Scotland convened a workshop to consider how the nursing professions could prepare themselves to take on the challenges arising from rapidly changing forces in health care. The hundred or so participants were preregistration students, nurses, midwives and health visitors, all nominated by health boards, colleges of nursing and midwifery, universities, professional organisations and statutory bodies.

The eventual outcome was *A Strategy for Nursing, Midwifery and Health Visiting in Scotland* (Scottish Home and Health Department, 1990). A personal copy of this document was sent to the 65 000 and more nurses, midwives and health visitors then effectively registered in Scotland, whether or not they were in practice. The document was an agreed statement of the philosophy of the nursing professions in Scotland, encompassing beliefs, values and purpose together with key objectives that had to be worked towards so that these could be reflected in practice, management, education and research.

Two of the objectives were:

> to ensure that all staff have access, as required, to sources of professional and personal counselling.

> to ensure that standards of care are developed and monitored, and a system for nursing audit is established.

Strategy project

It was recognised that none of the key objectives in this strategy would be anything more than empty words unless translated into action plans, implemented and audited. Thus the strategy project was set up. Its purpose was to encourage nurses, midwives and health visitors in the NHS, independent and voluntary sectors, as individuals or groups, to use reflective practice and collegial working to develop action plans for the strategy objectives, implement these and assess their effect. A national project officer was appointed to facilitate this, with the help of a steering group.

Expressions of interest to participate in the strategy project were invited from nurses, midwives and health visitors in the NHS, the independent and voluntary sectors, and professional organisations. From bids received, 17 project groups were set up and supported over 18 months. During this time, national conferences were held to demonstrate progress made and to encourage similar activity across Scotland (Scottish Office Home and Health Department, 1991).

Audit project

Investment in developing nursing audit followed with the Scottish Nursing Audit Development Project. Funded by the Scottish Office, it was in operation from late 1993 to early 1996. Its focus was to establish database information on audit activities, to foster supportive networks and to offer facilitator help at national and local levels.

Distance learning project

To complement this, the distance learning programme *Moving to Audit* (University of Dundee Centre for Medical Education, 1994), was developed with funding from the Scottish Office. It consists of a resource book and a series of audit challenges and activities. In the period between the launch in March 1994 and May 1995, these were issued free of charge to the 12 000 or so individual practitioners who asked for them.

All those who completed each challenge and returned it to the University of Dundee received personalised feedback together with an anonymised breakdown of how others had responded. A certificate of completion was awarded to those who completed all six challenges and activities and returned them to the university.

Calls for clinical supervision

An explicit call for clinical supervision had been made to the NHS in Scotland in *The Post Registration Education of Nurses, Midwives and Health Visitors* (National Nursing and Midwifery Advisory Committee, 1992). This noted concern about the lack of appropriate courses of training for those acting as supervisors to post-registration students and about lack of funding to allow for replacement staff while such preparation was being undertaken.

The need for practice supervision and professional support was reiterated in *Health Service Developments and the Scope of Professional Nursing Practice* (Laurenson, 1995), a survey conducted for the National Nursing, Midwifery and Health Visiting Advisory Committee.

The nursing professions in Scotland were not party to the work in England that followed on from the tragedies in the Grantham and Kesteven paediatric unit. Nevertheless, there was an independent but parallel groundswell of interest and investment in improving care by providing support for professional development through reflective practice and nursing audit.

What is clinical supervision?

Collaboration

Through the generosity of the English NHSE Nursing Directorate, materials on clinical supervision sent out to Directors of Nursing Services in England were shortly afterwards issued to their Scottish counterparts. In May 1995, all Directors of Nursing Services were invited to bid for their Trust to become one of the five Scottish sites to be included in the 23-site clinical supervision evaluation study masterminded from the School of Nursing Studies at the University of Manchester (Butterworth *et al.*, 1997). This highlighted clinical supervision on the agenda of meetings between the Scottish Office Directorate of Nursing and the nursing professions.

Presentations in Scotland from 1994 onwards were made by Professors Bishop and Butterworth to meetings of practitioners, educators, researchers and managers of nursing services. These helped to shift thinking on from the compartmentalisation of preceptors (for preregistration support), supervisors (for post-registration practice) and mentors (for career choices or career progression considerations) to collective consideration of the convenience packaging offered by Proctor's 'all-the-eggs-in-one-basket' construct of clinical supervision (Proctor, 1991) as an amalgam of formative, normative and restorative components.

Understanding

However, away from the charismatic presence of these two professors, did we really have a shared idea of what clinical supervision was about? If we did, could it be expressed in plain English to make successful bids for funding to purseholding NHS Trust Chief Executives and their non-nursing executive and non-executive directors? For this chapter, it seemed important to check this out.

Two sources were used. First, there were the evaluation forms completed by some of the hundred from across the nursing professions who attended the national seminar held in Edinburgh in June 1996 entitled 'Staff Support Systems: Clinical Supervision and Complementary Approaches'. Second, there were the returns from a November 1996 survey conducted among a small group of post-registration students pursuing undergraduate studies at Glasgow Caledonian University.

Comments

Comments made on almost all of the evaluation forms returned by those who attended the June seminar were favourable, but 10 people took time to make it known that they, in the words of one of them:

> Felt cheated.

They had wanted and expected the day to be:

> Focused on the actual setting up and doing [of clinical supervision]

and on specifics like:

> The recommended amount of supervisees allocated to supervisors.

They had wanted more on clinical supervision evaluation. One respondent wrote:

> I regret that speakers majored on stress and identifying the need for clinical supervision rather than actually talking about clinical supervision,

going on to say that speakers:

> Discussed areas of support but did not actually speak about clinical supervision.

This was feedback on a programme that had included presentations on: research into the support needs of such differing groups as practice nurses and cancer nurses (Wilkinson, 1995); the 23-site clinical supervision evaluation study in progress in England and Scotland; the UKCC 1996 position paper (UKCC, 1996) on clinical supervision; and innovative ways of supporting clinical practice by the use of designated link nurses at Edinburgh Health Care NHS Trust (Nottingham and O'Neill, 1996) and the use of an interactive CD-ROM training package developed at Falkirk and District Royal Infirmary NHS Trust (Laurenson, 1995).

Such comments caused this author, the organiser, to re-examine her own interpretation of clinical supervision and to realise that it might be at odds with that of others directly engaged in trying to think through how to introduce it in their workplace.

Questionnaire

Given the usual constraints of time and money, it was decided to devise a short questionnaire and ask a small group of post-registration undergraduate students at Glasgow Caledonian University whether they would help by completing it. Twenty-five agreed to do so. Twenty-one of these described their work as being:

> largely clinical.

Eight said that they had a system of clinical supervision in place where they worked. A further six said that discussions about how, when and where to introduce it were presently in progress. Five said they had been formally designated as supervisors, and nine had been formally designated as a preceptor, mentor or staff counsellor at some time.

So one might have expected largely positive responses to the question 'Frankly, are you clear about what is meant by the term "clinical supervision"?' However only three said yes to this.

In response to the invitation 'If you have a clear idea of clinical supervision, please say what it is for you', they offered brief statements such as:

> Supervision of students/trained staff by an accredited supervisor.

> A system whereby a person has an allocated mentor to work with during clinical time.

> An opportunity to discuss caseload with peers/managers.

Fifteen ticked the 'not entirely clear' option and four ticked 'confused', but no-one ticked 'no idea'.

However, when invited to say what were likely to be the main benefits of clinical supervision to patients/clients, participating staff and their organisation as a whole, 16 offered positive statements such as:

Keeping own skills updated within own work setting with benefits to patients.

For staff it can be a way of evaluating their practice and of getting feedback. For patients, if a staff member is improving practice through this, it can only be good for them.

The patients will have the benefit of confident, supervised staff. Participating staff will be more confident and their practice will be assessed and updated.

It should allow better communications between staff, highlighting areas of practice which may need to be focused on.

For patients, alternative approaches to management can be discussed, for staff, some benefits and some disadvantages, for the organisation, the NHS likes audit and it will be a good selling point for purchasers.

Will pass on good techniques to others and maintain and improve standards.

It should enable the person being supervised to enhance skills and reflect on their clinical practice.

Standards are maintained and stress is perhaps reduced.

Teaching and support for all levels of staff ensuring practice is research based and so will improve patient care.

These responses on the benefits of clinical supervision seemed like good news. However, when contrasted with the replies to the earlier questions 'Are you clear as to what is meant by the term...?' and 'If you have a clear idea of clinical supervision, please say what it is', a growing suspicion was strengthened. Could it be that the discrete vocabulary of the educator used in the much-quoted Proctor (1991) construct deterred even enthusiasts from trying to repeat it or paraphrase it?

Hopes and hunger

In any event, these two different sources – the seminar evaluation forms and the small survey of post-registration under-graduates in one university – indicate high hopes for the impact of clinical supervision on patient care and suggest a real appetite for advice on the 'how to' of implementation and evaluation.

What is actually happening?

The Scottish Directors of Nursing Services Group agreed to contribute to this section. Nurses working in six diverse health care settings across Scotland not participating in the 23-site evaluation study (Butterworth *et al.*, 1997) were also invited to contribute. Four agreed to do so. The accounts of activity that they provided are the substance of the following section.

Action by the Scottish NHS Trust Directors of Nursing Services Group

Report

In October 1996, the Scottish NHS Trust Directors of Nursing Services (DNS) endorsed the report of their working group on clinical supervision (Scottish NHS Trust Directors of Nursing Services Group, 1996). This expressed concern that 'Professional and organisational needs were not being addressed in equal measure' in discussions on clinical supervision. For that reason, the working group had been formed: 'To explore the opportunities and challenges both for nurses and their employers' presented by clinical supervision. Taking the headings of professional issues, education, management and research from the Scottish Strategy (Scottish Home and Health Department, 1990) it had considered how clinical supervision might impact on these areas.

Definition

The definition of clinical supervision used by the working group was:

> a planned exchange between professionals to enable the development of expertise which will enhance the delivery of care.

Benefits

The working group agreed that reasons for establishing and maintaining systems of supervision must be grounded in arguments firmly focused on improvement in the quality of patient care. They believed that this would attract greater support for the adoption of clinical supervision from both within and outside the nursing professions.

Benefits that the working group envisaged clinical supervision could deliver for patient care 'should occur through enhanced support and validation of professional activities by a professional peer, a peer group or an expert', but their report warned that claims to benefits for patient care would require to be tested through objective evaluation.

They saw that clinical supervision should reduce the gap between theory and practice. For this to happen, supervisors would have to have a sound, theory-based understanding of the processes of nursing: 'Through the sharing of this understanding clinical supervision should assist the practitioner to reflect upon the content and process of their practice.'

For the DNS group, clinical supervision should follow directly from preregistration preceptorship and, in doing so, support achievement of the UKCC requirements for post-registration continuing education.

Management

While acknowledging that the UKCC position statement (UKCC, 1996) said that supervision should not be the overt exercise of managerial responsibility or managerial supervision, the DNS group believed that 'There could still be scope to harmonise the more formal measurement of performance with the support that clinical supervision should offer.'

Costs

On costs, their report stated that 'Supervision cannot be cost neutral. It involves both time and skills.' Examples of costs were those incurred in: preparing and agreeing a credible model of supervision; training for supervisors; preparation time for all parties concerned to ensure that supervision sessions were properly planned and structured; time to fulfil commitments arising from supervision; and the loss of service provision to patients or clients while these activities were being pursued.

As to risk management, clinical supervision was seen as a means of reducing risk to patients and clients through ensuring that practice was evidence based.

Stress

Their report found that there was conflicting evidence surrounding the issue of stress levels in nurses and their effects. It was nevertheless of the view that supervision might play a significant part in ensuring that normal stress was met with support and prevented from developing into distress and consequent dysfunction, which may in turn 'draw a Trust into a position of vicarious liability'.

Imperatives

The report concluded by listing 11 imperatives for those seeking to implement clinical supervision sensitively and safely:

1 Ensure that the support of the Trust is available to implement and maintain appropriate systems of supervision.
2 Ensure that nurses who undertake complex clinical casework and those delivering their skills in isolated circumstances, either through remote geography or complex organisational structures, are offered the opportunity to receive supervision.
3 Ensure that the continuing development of skills and knowledge through lifelong learning is facilitated following preceptorship.
4 Aim toward research topics relevant to practice being discussed during supervision.

5 Ensure that supervision is considered in tandem with models of performance evaluation where appropriate.
6 Ensure that adequate training and support is available for supervisors.
7 Ensure that clear guidelines are developed for the implementation and evaluation of supervision.
8 Aim to measure the value added to patient care through supervision.
9 Ensure that protocols exist to allow supervisees to change supervisor where appropriate.
10 Consider engaging the support of academic institutions when seeking to evaluate the benefits from any supervision model.
11 Ensure that the costs of establishing models of supervision are fully evaluated.

Action by Shetland Health Board

Sandra Laurenson, Chief Nursing Adviser and Director of Service Development at Shetland Health Board, reports for this chapter that, following the results of a 1995 audit by questionnaire of the amount and type of support available to nursing staff and the subsequent publication of the UKCC position statement (UKCC,1996), it was felt that there was a need to address the provision of clinical supervision for staff in the Shetland Health Board directly managed unit.

Policy

To do this, she and all the senior nurse managers and nurse educators met together in a group facilitated by the quality co-ordinator. This group produced a policy for clinical supervision that presented staff with a variety of options in relation to selection of supervisor, number of supervisees per supervisor, method of supervision and frequency of supervision sessions.

The group felt that it was important not to be too prescriptive owing to the fact that supervision needs vary. They also recognised the fact that their policy had to cover junior as well as senior staff working within both hospital and community settings. The diverse geography of the Shetland Isles also meant that the policy had to encompass what would be possible for sole nurses working within isolated non-doctor settings as well as for those working in the hospital wards.

Pilots

Having produced the policy, it was decided to pilot it in various areas representative of nursing in Shetland. The areas selected were acute inpatient surgery, long-term care of the elderly with dementia and community nursing.

The pilot studies were to run for 5 months. At that point, a formal evaluation of the clinical supervision system would be carried out. Any problems identified would be addressed then and, should it be necessary, appropriate amendments be made to the policy.

Providing that no major unforeseen problems arise, the clinical supervision policy will be implemented gradually across the Shetland Hospitals and Community Services Unit.

Questionnaire

The questionnaire used in 1995 to collect staff views on the strengths and shortcomings of arrangements then in place for staff support is to be used again 1 year after the introduction of the clinical supervision system. This will allow staff views on the new system to be compared with their views on what existed before clinical supervision was in place.

Guidance

The 1996 Shetland guidance may be helpful to others in drawing up documents for their own situation, so extracts from it are given below:

Aims

In bringing practitioners and skilled supervisors together to reflect on practice, clinical supervision aims to identify solutions to problems, improve practice and increases understanding of professional issues. This corresponds to the goals of clinical supervision as identified by Platt-Koch (1986):

- To expand the practitioners' knowledge base.
- To assist in developing clinical proficiency.
- To develop autonomy and self-esteem as a professional.

Clinical supervision should build upon the support and assistance provided to newly registered practitioners via preceptorship.

While clinical supervision is aimed at clinical practitioners, locally this will be extended to cover colleagues in educational and managerial settings.

Rights and responsibilities

The rights and responsibilities of supervisees and supervisors are set out as follows. For the *supervisee*:

All supervisees will be given the opportunity to self-select their supervisor and to negotiate with them their preferred model of clinical supervision from the options available.

Supervisees in Shetland are asked to send notification of the selected supervisor by a specified date to their DNS, and, to make it easy for them to do this, a form is attached to the copy of the clinical supervision guidance given to each member of staff.

The guidance goes on to say:

Upon commencement of employment all new members of staff will be informed of the procedure for notifying the Director of Nursing Services of their chosen clinical supervisor.

Supervisees should identify practice issues for exploring and improve their ability to share these issues, explore interventions that are useful, be open to feedback and develop an ability to discriminate between helpful and unhelpful feedback.

The Shetland guidance on the rights and responsibilities of *supervisors* includes the following:

A supervisor is a practitioner who is skilled and experienced within the particular area of practice. It is anticipated that supervisors will be of the same grade or a higher grade than that of the supervisee.

The supervisee self-selecting the supervisor should help to facilitate the development of an effective professional supervisory relationship between the two individuals.

Supervisors should establish a safe environment for supervision, identifying clear boundaries for the session. They should explore and clarify thinking, giving clear feedback when required. It is the responsibility of supervisors to share their experience and skills and to confront personal and professional blocks while being aware of the relevant organisational issues.

Where the supervisory relationship also reflects the management hierarchy, it is vital for supervisors to remember that clinical supervision and their management function are two discrete entities and thus no confusion of the two will occur. As clinical supervision is being extended to cover all registered nurses in the unit, it is acknowledged that supervision at certain levels may be provided by members of other professional groups.

While it is the responsibility of each supervisor to decide how many supervisees he or she can supervise, it is envisaged that supervisors will have no more than four supervisees in order to enable the maximum benefit to be gained from clinical supervision while minimising the impact on the workload of the supervisor. In the case of group supervision, these arrangements will vary.

Models

Models preferred in Shetland were:
- one-to-one supervision from within the profession;
- one-to-one supervision with a supervisor from another discipline;
- one-to-one peer supervision with the supervisor being an individual of similar grade and expertise;
- peer group supervision, in which supervision is shared by members of the peer group. For these meetings, a designated facilitator should be identified from within the group, this role being rotated amongst group members.

While there are no formal links between clinical supervision and the appraisal of performance system used throughout the Shetland Hospitals and Community Services Unit, it is expected that supervision sessions will highlight personal development needs that will then be reflected in the performance appraisal system. If personal development needs have been identified, it is the supervisee's responsibility to negotiate appropriate options with the line manager.

It is anticipated that supervision sessions should occur at least quarterly, the exact arrangements being agreed between supervisor and supervisee.

Support and education for supervisors

As it is recognised that clinical supervision places additional responsibility on supervisors, adequate support mechanisms are to be made available to them. This will be in the form of an open-door policy whereby supervisors can approach the quality co-ordinator or another member of staff of their choice at any time for support or to discuss issues of concern while maintaining the individual supervisee's confidentiality.

In order to enable the supervisors to undertake their role properly, appropriate education is to be available. Courses held by the education and training department will cover issues such as the principles of supervision and communication skills, thus enabling the supervisor to assist supervisees in reflecting on their practice and to facilitate the learning process.

Documentation

In Shetland, documentation of supervision sessions is to take the following form:

- the supervisor should notify the line manager of the frequency and length of supervision sessions (a form is provided for this);
- supervisees should make a note of the content of sessions, for example in their personal profile.

It must be remembered that wherever details of the supervision are recorded that an individual's right to confidentiality must be maintained at all times.

A computerised record of supervisees and their supervisors will be kept by the Director of Nursing Services.

Annually each supervisee will be asked to sign and return a proforma to certify that they have had access to, and received, the clinical supervision that they required.

Action by West Lothian NHS Trust

West Lothian NHS Trust offers a wide spectrum of general acute, psychiatric, midwifery and community nursing services just outside Edinburgh, together with the regional burns, plastics and maxillofacial service for the east of Scotland. Libby Campbell, as Director of Nursing and Quality, provided the following information on the Trust's use of supervision contracts and mix of collegial and hierarchical systems for this chapter.

Strategy

As part of the 1996 Strategy for Nursing within West Lothian Trust, clinical supervision is highlighted as an area of practice development. The Strategy states that:

Every nurse will have access to a clinical supervisor so that they have the opportunity to discuss their individual clinical practice in a mutually beneficial environment.

There are three subheadings below this objective: the need to identify an appropriate system for the nursing specialty concerned so that it meets its philosophy; the educational needs of staff involved will be identified and met; and the system will be audited after 12 months.

Models

Each of the directorates within the Trust and each of the specialties within the directorates has been free to develop models appropriate to their specialties, while midwives have continued the established model for midwife supervision.

Clinical supervision agreement

Within mental health areas, for example, a clinical supervision agreement is reached between each practitioner and supervisor, setting out their shared objectives along with the time commitment for both and identifying the potential difficulties envisaged. In the main, the supervisors have emerged as the charge nurses for all ward staff and the line manager for the staff above charge nurse level. Within the community psychiatric nursing service, the supervisor is the directorate nurse manager. Evaluation will be carried out in due course, but initial indications are good.

Supervision contract

The model chosen for use in the intensive care area is that of peer group support; this is conducive to an area that is staffed with a high ratio of qualified staff at higher grades. In practice, this also involves a 'supervision contract', but this is overridden as required if, for example, there is need to discuss a specific situation that has occurred or to talk to non-nursing staff as well. Evaluation will also take place here. Indications so far are also good.

Action by Greater Glasgow Community and Mental Health Services NHS Trust

The system for identifying supervisors devised by Greater Glasgow Community and Mental Health Services NHS Trust is especially interesting. From this setting, Karen Lockhart, as

Senior Nurse (Projects), tells us in her own words about the approach to clinical supervision adopted there.

> As one of the largest Trusts in Britain with around 2500 nursing staff, the task of implementing clinical supervision is a considerable challenge. Staff express great enthusiasm for the introduction of clinical supervision as they feel they have greater responsibility and autonomy than ever before and would like some sort of safety net to support them.

Models

Various forms of 'supervision' are, in fact, already ongoing. One example is that of the outpatient adolescent psychiatry nursing team who have had clinical supervision for some years. Supervision in this setting is a process of regular case review between the practitioner and the line manager who holds ultimate responsibility for case management. The purpose is:

- To provide the practitioner with an opportunity for training and development;
- To ensure quality in clinical practice.

Supervision can take the form of a case discussion, screening and reviewing videotapes. The objective is to train psychiatric nurses in therapeutic techniques, and to establish a process of review and supervision linked to a learning contract, to support the supervision of effective assessment and treatment, and regularly to review all patients currently receiving treatment.

Another example is a Mental Health Resource Centre, in which three community psychiatric nurses hold monthly supervision sessions. At each session, one of the community psychiatric nurses is the supervisee, one is supervisor and one acts as a consultant to the supervisor. The roles are rotated at each session, so each community psychiatric nurse has an hour of supervision every 3 months. This group periodically invites a psychiatrist to sit in to evaluate how its members are performing. They feel this helps them to avoid some of the traps they could fall into as three peers supervising each other, such as blinkered perspectives and being overly empathetic.

Steering group

The process of introducing clinical supervision across the Trust was launched with a seminar of invited speakers from elsewhere who had already developed clinical supervision, and from the UKCC. This was attended by approximately 150 staff and was followed by group sessions for each discipline to discuss the perceived requirements of clinical supervision and allow staff input into the evaluation process.

Volunteers from the seminar formed a steering group which is responsible for implementing pilot sites across the Trust. This group was given access to a collection of 36 articles on clinical supervision and asked to choose the ones which they would like to read to prepare themselves for their forthcoming role. This helped to give the group confidence, especially those members who had had no formal experience of clinical supervision.

Definition

This steering group chose a working definition for supervision that allows the continuation of existing models of good practice but does not set too high a standard for new sites. This definition is:

> Clinical supervision should be practice focused; empower clients and patients; make a significant contribution to helping purchasers and providers of health care discuss and share practice; sustain and develop practice; and contain explicit outcomes for patients and practitioners.

Supervisors

The group next agreed the skills and attributes that would be required in a supervisor, including:

- in-depth, up-to-date knowledge of the specialty;
- at least 2 years' 'on-the-job' experience;
- to be currently in clinical practice.

It is intended that staff will nominate colleagues whom they feel have these attributes. Thus the pool of supervisors in the Trust will have been chosen by their peers, although individual supervisees will not choose the particular supervisor allocated to them.

Pilots

The group then set about deciding which form the pilots should take. It was thought necessary to test various types of supervision in the different settings across the Trust. An evaluation strategy will be developed which will be applied to all sites. This evaluation will include a costing element because there is a belief that group supervision is less expensive than one-to-one supervision. It will be important to test whether this is, in fact, the case.

The plan is to adopt the Proctor view (1991) that clinical supervision should fulfil three functions: formative, restorative and normative. The models to be piloted are one-to-one supervision, group supervision with a designated supervisor and group supervision with a rotating supervisor.

Throughout the various functional areas of the Trust, the intention is to introduce clinical supervision in these three forms. For example, three community bases will introduce clinical supervision for health visiting, one using the 'one-to-one' model, one using the group with designated supervisor model and one using the group with each health visitor taking a turn at being supervisor. Each of these will be evaluated. The evaluation will look for evidence that health visitors feel adequately supported and can demonstrate development of knowledge. Likewise, mental health inpatient wards will pilot all three models and have an evaluation carried out.

This will test the efficacy of the three chosen models and allow their effect and cost to be compared.

Action by Lanarkshire Education Providers

Preparation

The preparation of supervisors in one Trust is described from an education provider's perspective. Marie Cerinus, Senior Lecturer at Bell College of Technology, writes the following section.

At the beginning of 1995, Lanarkshire College of Nursing and Midwifery, now part of the School of Nursing and Midwifery of Bell College of Technology, was delighted to receive a request from a local NHS Trust to collaborate in the preparation of selected groups of nurses for the introduction of clinical supervision. In undertaking this work, the College was able to build upon a long-established relationship with the nurses of that Trust, a relationship that had been consolidated over the preceding 3 years in the preparation and support of nurses for the preceptorship of preregistration students.

Preparation for preceptorship had demanded, as a minimum, the provision of a 5-day course, underpinning which was the value of professional support for continuous professional development, support provided by preceptors for their preceptees, and the managerial and educational support provided by care area managers and college lecturers for the preceptors themselves.

Within the preceptorship preparation, the key elements of clinical supervision, self-awareness, reflection, reflective practice and teaching–learning relationships had already been established as the essential elements of professional support and development. Therefore, with the fundamentals necessary to the successful implementation of clinical supervision already established through preceptorship preparation, and subsequently developed through the practice and support of preceptorship, they were now ready for application to another context. This context is one of a formalised professional support mechanism for all practitioners – clinical supervision.

Definition

The definition of clinical supervision adopted by the Trust was:

> a formal process of professional support and learning which enables individual practitioners to develop knowledge and competence, assume responsibility for their own practice and enhance consumer protection and the safety of care in complex clinical situations. (Department of Health, 1993)

Sessions

In keeping with this definition and the Trust's own project plan and protocol for clinical supervision, the College planned and delivered five separate teaching sessions aimed at different groups of nurses, depending on their role within the Trust. Essentially, all the nurses identified by the Trust to participate in the launch of clinical supervision, including immediate line managers, received some form of preparation. This was to emphasise the absolute need for managers and nurses to have a shared understanding of clinical supervision to facilitate its effective implementation.

These sessions, as well as providing essential information about the Trust's strategy on clinical supervision, were also designed to encourage exploration of its conceptual basis and the means of introducing this professional support mechanism. Through this active involvement in the preparatory process, a shared appreciation of the value of clinical supervision to professional practice and its development could evolve, in addition to a sense of ownership.

Given the demands that nurses face, it was also felt important to provide time within these preparatory sessions to enable the nurses to produce an action plan for implementing clinical supervision within their own areas. This gave explicit recognition to the varied contexts within which nurses work, each one of which demands a discrete plan of action. It also ensured that clinical supervision was not imposed from a purely theoretical or strategical management perspective. To be successful, clinical supervision must meet the needs of those it is designed to serve: the nurses themselves. They must therefore be active in its establishment, albeit with the support of strategic management and based on sound theoretical underpinnings.

Three other points were emphasised within these preparatory sessions. First, that clinical supervision cannot be viewed as an extension of, nor a substitute for, managerial supervision. Second, clinical supervision is not a panacea for all ills: it does not compensate for the ineffective provision and management of resources. Third, because clinical supervision reflects the reality of nursing practice, focusing as it does on care delivery, its problems, solutions and development, it demands rigour and commitment to be effective and therefore cannot be undertaken lightly.

Guidelines

Throughout this preparation for clinical supervision, the College and Trust's collaborative effort attempted to encapsulate the spirit and practicality of the guidelines compiled by Kohner (1994), which identify the following essentials:

1 Establish a clear definition of and purpose for clinical supervision.
2 Involve all in the planning and implementation of clinical supervision.
3 Give careful consideration to the qualifications, skills and experience required in supervisors.
4 Ensure appropriate training that focuses on the skills of supervision.
5 Provide supervision for supervisors to develop the quality of supervision.
6 Make supervision available to all practitioners, regardless of seniority.
7 Set clear boundaries for the content and process of supervision.
8 Formally constitute ground rules for supervision relationships.
9 Agree on evaluation methods for clinical supervision.
10 Provide sustained organisational commitment to clinical supervision.

All of these guidelines were addressed within the preparatory sessions.

Value

On reflection, the value of delivering only preparatory sessions must be questioned. Clinical supervision demands lifelong commitment to professional learning and development if it is to enhance patient and client care. Therefore, lifelong support is needed in addition to the initial preparation. Just as preceptorship continues to flourish through preparation and ongoing support, so would clinical supervision.

Conclusion

These snapshots of activity in Scotland illustrate something of the interest in clinical supervision. There is real commitment to use the opportunities presented by the present spotlight on clinical supervision to help nurses and health visitors to improve their practice and, through this, the care they give to patients and clients.

Audit

The Shetland Health Board approach seems to offer a model for anyone who has to devise and implement an action plan for the introduction of clinical supervision for no matter which specialty. It used the results of an audit of available staff support as the starting point. Senior nurses then agreed a policy for using clinical supervision to make good deficits that this audit identified. This policy encompasses arrangements for the key elements of a clinical supervision system. It gives a list of processes and anticipated outcomes that can be audited, adjusted if necessary and audited again. Overall evaluation of the benefit of clinical supervision to staff will be assessed through a repeat of the questionnaire audit used before the introduction of clinical supervision.

Ownership

The strength of the approach of the Greater Glasgow Community and Mental Health Services NHS Trust, with its large workforce, is that it devised a way of giving a sense of ownership of the system to its employees. To do this, it set about recruiting staff interest and support, with high-profile investment of time and energy, in involving the potential supervisees in formulating the processes to be used in their clinical supervision. The approach used for the selection of supervisors is particularly interesting since it charged volunteer members of the supervisee group with deciding the criteria that supervisors should meet. These having been agreed by the potential supervisees, the allocation of supervisors to supervisees is then the job of management.

Managers as supervisors

Supervision contracts or agreements are used in all of the pilots at West Lothian NHS Trust. It may be that these prove to be useful mechanisms for helping supervisors who are also line managers to separate their supervisory relationship from their management function. To purists, it is not appropriate that line managers should be directly engaged in clinical supervision, but in the real world the issue of manager-as-supervisor is a live one. Indeed, staff within mental health areas in West Lothian NHS Trust have themselves chosen to have line managers as their supervisors. In other areas of the Trust used as pilot sites, supervisors are peer group members. Time and the outcome of evaluation studies will tell whether the manager-as-supervisor option is workable.

Preparation and support

The importance of appropriate preparation and continuing support for supervisors is mentioned at several points in this chapter. The Lanarkshire approach offers a starting point for those trying to set this up and examine possible costs. There would certainly seem to be a case to be made for examining how preparation and continuing support might be offered in a way that builds on previous preparation for preceptorship where this has already been undertaken.

Future developments

The report of the DNS group (Scottish NHS Trust Directors of Nursing Services Group, 1996) will influence further developments in clinical supervision in Scotland, as will the findings from the 23-site evaluation study by Manchester University (Butterworth *et al.*, 1997)

It is to be hoped that the outcomes of the evaluations conducted by the contributors to this chapter will be shared as they become available via the nursing press for the benefit of us all.

The activity described here has yet to be weathered over time, its products evaluated and its processes costed. However, the different examples given of how clinical supervision has been introduced should be helpful to others thinking about using it in their place of work.

References

Butterworth, T., Carson, J., White, E., Jeacock, J., Clements, A. and Bishop, V. 1997 *It Is Good to Talk. An Evaluation of Clinical Supervision and Mentorship in England and Scotland*. Manchester: University of Manchester School of Nursing and Midwifery.

Department of Health 1993 *A Vision for the Future. The Nursing, Midwifery and Health Visiting Contribution to Health and Health Care*. London: HMSO.

Kohner, N. 1994 *Clinical Supervision in Practice*. London: King's Fund Centre.

Laurenson, S., for the National Nursing, Midwifery and Health Visiting Advisory Committee 1995 *Health Service Developments and the Scope of Professional Nursing Practice: A Survey of Developing Roles within NHS Trusts in Scotland*. Edinburgh: National Professional Advisory Committees' Secretariat.

National Nursing and Midwifery Advisory Committee 1992 *The Post-registration Education of Nurses, Midwives and Health Visitors*.

Report of a Working Group (Chair: Professor M.F. Alexander). Edinburgh: Scottish Office Home and Health Department.

Nottingham, C. and O'Neill, F. 1996 *Report of the Strengthening Cancer Care 1995–96 Initiative*. Edinburgh: Scottish Office.

Platt-Koch, L.M 1986 Clinical supervision for psychiatric nurses. *Journal of Psycho-social Nursing* **26**(1): 7–15.

Proctor, B. 1991 Supervision: a cooperative exercise in accountability. In: Marken, M. and Payne, M. (eds) *Enabling and Ensuring: Supervision in Practice*. Leicester: National Youth Bureau and Council for Education and Training in Youth and Community Work.

Scott, P.H. 1985 *In Bed with an Elephant*. Edinburgh: Saltire Society.

Scottish Home and Health Department 1990 *A Strategy for Nursing, Midwifery and Health Visiting in Scotland*. Edinburgh: HMSO.

Scottish NHS Trust Directors of Nursing Services Group 1996 *Clinical Supervision: Report of the Director of Nursing Services Working Group* (Chair: R. Brown). Lochgilphead: Argyll and Bute NHS Trust Headquarters.

Steering Group for the Strategy for Nursing, Midwifery and Health Visiting in Scotland 1991 *Interim Report*. Edinburgh: Scottish Office Home and Health Department.

UKCC (United Kingdom Central Council for Nursing, Midwifery and Health Visiting) 1996 *Position Statement on Clinical Supervision for Nursing and Health Visiting*. London: UKCC.

University of Dundee Centre for Medical Education 1994 *Moving to Audit: An Educational Package for Nurses, Midwives and Health Visitors*. Dundee: Centre for Medical Education.

Wilkinson, S.M. 1995 The changing pressures for cancer nurses 1986–93. *European Journal of Cancer Care*, **4**: 69–74.

5

Clinical Supervision: Its Implementation in one Acute Sector Trust

Chrissy Dunn and Veronica Bishop

This chapter describes in detail how clinical supervision was set up, using an 'opting in' process in a large acute Trust spread across two sites. Initial discussions with colleagues indicated that knowledge of the subject was varied, as was the interest in it. Led by the practice development unit, information was 'snowballed' across the two sites, and the local university became involved in training needs. Supported by management, the concept of clinical supervision is growing in appeal, and clinical staff are developing appropriate expertise and evaluative systems to ensure its effective delivery.

Introduction

The changes made to the organisation and management of care within the NHS during recent years, and the impact that these changes have had on front-line staff such as nurses, is well documented in Chapter 1. The additional effects of the Clothier report (HMSO, 1995) and the DoH document *A Vision for the Future* (Department of Health, 1993) set in train local and national initiatives to explore and test the value of clinical supervision, a concept supported in principle by the UKCC and written into the business plans for 1993–97 and by the Royal College of Nursing (Royal College of Nursing, 1996).

The UKCC later ratified their approval of clinical supervision in the position statement of 1996.

The Trust, which has over 800 beds on two sites, and a high turnover level of patients with an average stay of under 5 days, currently employs around 1000 qualified nurses, who work in a wide range of clinical settings and within teams of varying size, skill mix and discipline. Two years ago, in response to the 'Vision' document (Department of Health, 1993), and in keeping with the Trust's value statement of 'People matter', clinical supervision was discussed informally by the senior practice development nurse, her team and the Trust Nurse Executive. The lead practice nurse was particularly motivated in her drive to introduce clinical supervision to the Trust as she felt that nurses needed to be supported in their work if they were to develop their practice while constantly responding to the needs of patients and colleagues. 'Pit-head' time – that time claimed by British coal miners to wash off the grime of the job in the boss's time (Hawkins and Shohet, 1992) – was, in her view, the right of every nurse. She shared the conviction with her Trust Nurse Executive that it 'paid off' in terms of improved patient care if nurses had time to stop and think about what they were doing and to reflect on their practice. The practice development nurses often used guided reflection techniques in their dealings with nurses and provided a confidential listening ear whenever necessary. However, clinical supervision offered a framework to formalise and improve on these aspects and to help nurses consider, in a safe environment, a range of issues, from ethical dilemmas and decision-making in a multiprofessional team, to innovative practices.

Getting clinical supervision on the Trust agenda

Considerable thought was given to how to set about introducing clinical supervision. Discussions with colleagues across the two hospital sites indicated that some nurses knew a little about the subject, although midwives had a particular understanding of it as it was part of their statutory requirement. Other staff, including department managers, showed a varying level of interest, and it must be said that not all were initially as enthusiastic as were the practice development nurses.

In order to establish the interest and commitment to clinical supervision, the practice development team held a study day to which a small number of each grade of nurse were invited, along with a nurse manager. While the day was fairly informal, the meeting was semistructured to ensure that the organiser's aims were met. It was essential to establish whether there was a wish to implement clinical supervision in the Trust. The practice development team was anxious to avoid clinical supervision being seen as a management tool or something being pushed from the top down. The purpose of the day was to explore openly the concept of clinical supervision and to discuss the implications for nurses and nursing practice in the Trust.

A dozen nurses attended the meeting, representing all grades, and the group was facilitated by two members of the practice development team. Questions addressed during the day included: Who should be clinical supervisors? What preparation do they need? How do we get up and running? How should clinical supervision be organised? Is it achievable? What are the risks and the benefits? How much will it cost? Not everyone was optimistic about the chances of introducing clinical supervision, and nurses, being in the main very pragmatic people, were conscious of the danger of promising something that could not be delivered. The 'think tank', as it became known, produced a written summary of its discussions that was circulated to all ward sisters for further discussion with their staff.

Organising clinical supervision

As a result of this exploratory work, the practice development team gained a clear impression of how nurses in the Trust viewed clinical supervision and how it could work out in practice. Essentially, nurses saw clinical supervision as a good way of developing their professional lives and improving patient care. The formative, restorative and normative functions of clinical supervision, adapted from Proctor (1991), were thought to be an appropriate foundation for any model(s) developed in the Trust. The majority of nurses believed that all trained staff working in clinical practice should have the opportunity to access clinical supervision following on after the 6-month preceptorship period for newly qualified staff, although this should not be made a condition of employment. Choice was a very important principle, and a strong preference was expressed that nurses should be able to *opt in*, rather than opt out, of clinical supervision, both as supervisees and supervisors. In addition, nurses wanted to be able to choose their supervisor from an approved list of specially prepared, experienced practitioners.

Suggested frequency, time, venue and ground rules for sessions

The 'think tank' unanimously agreed that sessions should be one to one, in a private area, preferably at some distance from patients and telephone interruptions. They stressed that sessions should be booked in advance, generally for 1 hour, and that this should be protected time. Experience had taught staff that there was a tendency for other issues to take priority over staff needs, and it was therefore recognised as important to have the support of management and other clinical staff. It was thought possible to provide individual staff with clinical supervision every 6–8 weeks, and the suggestion was made that extra sessions could be arranged if necessary.

There was some disagreement on the most appropriate method of recording sessions, although all agreed that some degree of record-keeping was important. Confidentiality was also an issue discussed, as was the need to report malpractice should it come to light. It was agreed that guidelines should be designed for the Trust which would take these issues into account, and it was further recommended that supervisors be in supervision themselves. There was agreement that individual nurses should be able to select their supervisor, this person being seen as clinically credible and up to date with current practice.

Next steps: the cascade

Following the 'think tank', it was proposed that a staged programme of clinical supervision should be implemented in the Trust and its effectiveness evaluated over 1 year. The implementation should be managed by a 'cascade effect'. This could be achieved by selecting a small number of nurses (around 10) who were willing to train and act as supervisors. It was intended that, once trained, supervisors would have their names entered in a directory of clinical supervisors for the Trust and that this directory would be made available to nurses seeking supervision. After making their selection, the onus would be on the nurses seeking clinical supervision to approach the supervisor with the intention of agreeing a regular commitment to clinical supervision. The supervisor would also, of course, have the option to decline. It was thought quite likely that some supervisors would be particularly popular. Thus, to prevent individuals becoming victims of their own success, it was thought sensible to limit to three the number of supervisees for any one supervisor. The first nurses to train as supervisors were the five practice development nurses, four ward sisters and a clinical nurse specialist. Although this may appear to be a hierarchical move, the practice development nurses were not managerially accountable for any clinical staff. Also, as the practice development nurses enjoyed a collegial relationship with nurses in clinical areas, it was hoped that any 'top down' reservations would be negated.

Because of the reservations expressed in the 'think tank' that the term 'supervision' was misleading, and could even put staff off considering clinical supervision, introductory study days were organised. These continue to run three times a year and are funded through the practice development service. On these study days, the concept and functions of clinical supervision are explained, and a role play is enacted by two members of the practice development team. This role play focuses on a quite ordinary example of nursing practice, which is discussed between the 'supervisor' and 'supervisee'. The ordinariness of the incident, which produces important learning points for the 'supervisee', often surprises staff attending the introductory study day. There is a tendency to imagine that only extraordinary crisis situations get taken to clinical supervision. At the end of the introductory day, written information is supplied and the nurses are invited to contact their practice development nurse for a 'no obligation – free sample' of clinical supervision before committing themselves to a more permanent arrangement.

Starting the cascade: training supervisors

Discussion with nurse educators and practitioners, along with review of the literature, suggested that the programme of preparation for supervisors should include interpersonal skills required by clinical supervisors and the use of reflective practice. It was also thought important to include relevant professional, legal and ethical issues, and to provide participants with the opportunity to reflect on their personal experience as a supervisee.

With help from the department of nursing studies at the local university, a training programme for supervisors was devised, funding being made available by virement from existing budgets. The programme consists of a 2-day workshop and three follow-up sessions over a 3-month period. Entry criteria for the supervisors programme requires participants to be receiving regular clinical supervision themselves. They also need to have the support of their line manager both to attend the workshop and to act as a supervisor following its completion. Prior to the workshop, participants are given a pre-workshop pack containing a reading list, workshop programme and instructions on completing preparatory work prior to the workshop. The preparatory work asks the participant to select and write a short account of a critical incident from practice that they feel able to share with a colleague during the workshop. The second day of the workshop focuses on skills acquisition for the supervisor's role, and participants have particularly valued the opportunity to practise supervision skills, using the prepared critical incidents, in a safe and supportive environment.

The workshops are designed around the need to be familiar with the agreed elements of clinical supervision: those of support, education and standard-setting. There are sessions on recognising and responding to occupational stress, and time to explore the qualities needed by clinical supervisors. Ethical and professional dimensions of clinical supervision are also discussed. Further work centres on frameworks for reflective practice, and, as well as practising supervision skills, participants have the opportunity to meet experienced clinical supervisors and ask questions about the role. At the end of the workshop, arrangements for the three follow-up sessions are discussed and other information is given on practical matters such as finding rooms for supervision, the supervisors' directory and updating professional profiles.

With the first supervisors for the Trust prepared, 10 newly fledged (and rather nervous!) clinical supervisors put themselves forward to colleagues seeking clinical supervision. Within a few months, each had reached their full quota of supervisees, and there was also a waiting list of people wanting to attend future supervisors' workshops. Hence, during the next 2 years, we saw steady progress made on the availability of supervisors and the number of nurses accessing regular clinical supervision. A cascade of clinical supervision activity ensued as supervisees prepared to become supervisors. The enthusiastic take-up of places on the introductory study day encouraged us that the demand was stronger than ever, and we finally became convinced that we had a success on our hands.

However convincing all this might seem to those excited at the prospect of clinical supervision, we needed more concrete evidence if we were to persuade health care managers that clinical supervision was a good investment in terms of staff usage and improving patient care. For this reason, an evaluation programme was designed to run concurrently with the introduction of clinical supervision.

Evaluating clinical supervision

The objectives for the evaluation programme were:

- to determine whether the model of implementation provided a realistic and achievable framework for clinical supervision within the Trust;

- to assess the model's potential to facilitate the three components of clinical supervision: the supportive, educative and normative functions;
- to provide baseline data for future evaluation.

From the beginning, records were kept that would provide current information on clinical supervision activity taking place in the Trust. This included:

- the number of people acting as clinical supervisors;
- the number of people receiving clinical supervision;
- how often sessions were taking place;
- where sessions were being held;
- whether sessions were interrupted, cancelled or postponed;
- whether sessions were taking place in duty time;
- methods used to facilitate sessions and record proceedings.

By the end of the first year, 45 nurses had attended the supervisors' workshops, although at this stage 10 of these nurses had, for a variety of reasons including study and maternity leave, not yet commenced supervising nurses.

Sixty-three nurses were receiving regular clinical supervision within 22 wards and departments throughout the Trust. The average time between sessions was 5 weeks. It came as no surprise that one of the problems encountered by those engaging in clinical supervision was finding a quiet, private room conveniently close to the clinical areas to reach quickly but not so convenient that they were interrupted. In fact, at least a quarter of sessions were interrupted for one reason or another. A quarter had to be re-scheduled as service demands had required the session to be cancelled. Despite initial scepticism that clinical supervision would only happen in off-duty time, the majority of sessions took place while at least one of those concerned was on duty. Perhaps 'pit-head' time could become a reality after all. There was some initial concern that the sessions might become little more than time out for a chat and a cup and coffee. However, the results of evaluation at this stage suggested that over 90 per cent of clinical supervision sessions had utilised one of the reflective frameworks offered during the workshop. Simple note-taking and personal reflective diaries were popular methods of recording a session, but there was a tendency not to stick to one method; instead, different approaches were tried and tested.

Considering the quite radical nature of clinical supervision, the challenges it presented to nurses and managers alike, and the increasing demands being placed on time and energy, the results of clinical supervision activity occurring at this stage were better than expected. The results speak volumes for the sustained commitment of nurses engaging in clinical supervision (as well as those who enabled their colleagues to participate) and health care managers with the vision and foresight to support the work in its early stages.

Evaluating the supportive function

Sickness and absence

There is some belief that emotional well-being has an influence on sickness absence. For example, in 1988 the Health and Safety Executive estimated that up to 40 per cent of absenteeism could be a result of mental or emotional health problems (cited in Marshall, 1994). It was therefore decided to examine the amount of sickness and absence occurring in the wards using clinical supervision.

Figures were recorded for the 6-month period prior to clinical supervision and for a similar 6-month period following its introduction (Table 5.1).

Table 5.1   Number of days sickness absence taken by qualified staff

WARD	A	B	C	D	E	F	G
Number of days pre-clinical supervision (Sept 94–Feb 95)	119	83	349 (2 long-term sick)	145	160	159	102
Number of days post-clinical supervision (Sept 95–Feb 96)	41	106	76	104	98	275	182

Shaded areas indicates control wards.

Figures were also obtained for two wards not involved in clinical supervision. The number of days sickness and absence taken by nurses in the five pilot wards and two control wards indicated that there was a significant reduction in the number of days taken as sickness absence on four out of the five clinical supervision wards, whereas the two control wards had seen an increase in sickness absence taken by their nursing staff. This raises interesting questions on whether clinical supervision could have an impact on the general health of nurses.

Maslach burnout inventory

The emotional labour associated with nursing work has been well researched and reported (James, 1992; Smith, 1992). Butterworth *et al.* (1996) suggest a range of tools that could be used to measure degrees of occupational stress of nurses (see Chapter 8). In line with Butterworth's DoH-funded evaluation study (Butterworth *et al.*, 1997), all trained staff on two wards intending to introduce clinical supervision, and two control wards not planning to use clinical supervision, were asked to complete the adapted Maslach burnout inventory (Maslach and Jackson, 1981) at the beginning of the evaluation period to provide a baseline. The wards were matched for specialty and location on both hospital sites. Both sisters on the intervention wards had been prepared as clinical supervisors, and, during the next 12 months, a planned programme introduced clinical supervision to the team leaders and other key nurses within the nursing teams. At the end of this 12-month period, four nurses out of 14 on ward A, and nine nurses out of 18 on ward B, were engaging in clinical supervision. However, no clinical supervision activity had taken place on the two control wards. Average Maslach scores for all trained nurses on wards A, B, F and G were calculated pre- and post-clinical supervision. The average response rate for all the wards taking part was 86 per cent in 1995, and 42 per cent in 1996. Particularly acute staff shortages and high workloads were evident throughout the hospital during the time of administration of the questionnaire in 1996, which may have contributed to the low response rate.

Emotional exhaustion

The average pre and post scores on the emotional exhaustion subscale for the clinical supervision wards and two control wards for all four wards were within the moderate range at the beginning of the clinical supervision project. A year later, the average scores for the four wards were higher than previously, but for the two wards involved in clinical supervision the increase in score was slight. The two wards not involved in clinical supervision had a much greater increase in average score, taking both scores into the highly exhausted category (Table 5.2).

Table 5.2 Maslach burnout inventory results: emotional exhaustion subscale

1995 results:			
	Ward A	21.4	range 4–41
	Ward B	16.4	range 5–34
	Ward F	25.7	range 16–48
	Ward G	17.0	range 5–43
1996 results:			
	Ward A	23.2	range 13–47
	Ward B	16.7	range 4–37
	Ward F	31.6	range 16–45
	Ward G	30.0	range 11–48

Wards A and B = clinical supervision wards. Wards F and G = control wards.

Depersonalisation

The average pre and post scores on the depersonalisation subscale for the clinical supervision and control wards all fell within the moderate range (Table 5.3). One year later, the scores for the two wards involved in clinical supervision showed a slight drop that brought them into the 'OK' range. Of the wards not involved in clinical supervision, one showed a slight decrease within the moderate range of the depersonalisation scale, whereas another showed a significant increase that took staff from 'OK' to 'moderate' depersonalisation.

Table 5.3   Maslach scores: depersonalisation subscale

1995 results:				
	Ward A	7.1	range	0–27
	Ward B	4.17	range	0–15
	Ward F	8.7	range	1–23
	Ward G	3.7	range	0–11
1996 results:				
	Ward A	6.0	range	0–21
	Ward B	3.75	range	1–8
	Ward F	7.8	range	1–17
	Ward G	8.5	range	0–22

Wards A and B = clinical supervision wards. Wards F and G = control wards.

Personal accomplishment

The initial scores for all four wards were in the moderate or high burnout range (Table 5.4). One year later, the results for the clinical supervision and control wards indicate similar increases in personal accomplishment scores, taking one clinical supervision ward into the low burnout range.

Table 5.4   Maslach scores: personal accomplishment subscale

1995 results:				
	Ward A	33.0	range	24–40
	Ward B	34.4	range	14–46
	Ward F	29.1	range	12–41
	Ward G	34.0	range	21–45
1996 results:				
	Ward A	35.2	range	24–48
	Ward B	39.6	range	26–47
	Ward F	32.1	range	19–38
	Ward G	35.6	range	25–46

Wards A and B = clinical supervision wards. Wards F and G = control wards.

The reduction in the number of sickness absence days and the results of the Maslach inventory appear to indicate that staff working on wards where clinical supervision had been implemented fared better than those on the two control wards. However, it is important not to draw any firm conclusions from these results, especially when one considers the wide range of variables for which it would be impossible to control. As already stated, participation in the clinical supervision prog- ramme was entirely by choice, and it could be argued that staff keen to participate in such a scheme may have already recognised the need for systems of support or developed less formal strategies. During the implementation period, however, staff on all the wards were subjected to similar surges in service activity, organisational change and staffing difficulties. Although it would be worthwhile if wards undertook to repeat the exer- cise periodically to see whether any ongoing trends developed, it is perhaps unwise, and unfair, any longer to deny the control wards access to clinical supervision, especially as the staff are now keen to participate.

Evaluating the normative function

Nursing audit has been performed in all relevant clinical areas for the last 3 years using an in-house audit tool developed within the Trust. The audit, which takes place each year, is adminis- tered jointly by the ward sister, another nurse from outside the ward and the link tutor from the college. The audit tool generates a score in each of five sections, according to compli- ance with individual structure and process criteria:

- Nursing practice
- Manpower
- Management
- Staff development
- Learning environment

A percentage score is calculated in each section and an overall average score then calculated.

With the permission of the sisters on the wards taking part, it was decided to utilise these audit results to evaluate the possible effect of clinical supervision on the professional stan- dards of the ward. There is little or no difference between the pre and post overall nursing audit scores for any of the wards implementing clinical supervision, or for the two control wards, and this applied equally to scoring in the various sections. The exceptions were ward D, in which a contributing factor may have been a vacancy for a key member of staff during this period, and one of the control wards, which achieved a near-perfect score.

The use of this audit tool is currently under review within the Trust as, on reflection, it does not appear to be sensitive enough to establish a basis for changing practice. In addition, difficulties have arisen in ensuring consistency in its administration.

Evaluating the educative function

Clinical supervision is essentially an interpersonal process, and the practice development team was anxious to avoid falling into the trap of merely measuring what was measurable. We therefore needed to tackle the very real difficulties of evaluating personal experiences and learning effectiveness. To begin this process, we consulted our colleagues in nurse education, and a semistructured questionnaire was designed that asked supervisees to:

- describe their relationship with their supervisor;
- say whether or not their skill, knowledge and attitude to their work had changed as a result of clinical supervision, and, if it had to give an example;
- say what they liked most and least about their clinical supervision sessions.

Thirty-two questionnaires were returned by supervisees during the evaluation period, and content analysis has given us some fascinating insight into how the nurses viewed clinical supervision and the difference it made to their working lives.

How supervisees described the relationship with their supervisor

All respondents described their relationship with their supervisor in positive terms, especially the good feelings that they believed their relationship evoked. Supervisees needed to feel safe during clinical supervision, so they particularly valued a relationship with a supervisor for whom they felt respect and whom they could trust. Two respondents mentioned the dynamic nature of the relationship, which they said was developing over time, and two respondents felt that the relationship with the supervisor was crucial to the success of clinical supervision:

> I find it a comfortable relationship. It has been important for me to have a supervisor I have respect for and I value her opinion. I think the relationship between the supervisee and supervisor is the most important aspect in the success of clinical supervision. If the supervisee feels uncomfortable in the relationship, she is unlikely to be honest and the supervisor is unlikely to be honest.

Supervisees also described a number of personal qualities that they attributed to their supervisor. One third of respondents said that their clinical supervisor was a respected colleague, and clinical credibility was important to those in supervision as this led to equality and mutual respect. Respondents appreciated their supervisors being open and friendly, and supervisors with high personal integrity, who were honest, sincere and understanding, helped to create an environment in which difficult issues could safely be explored. Respondents also highlighted the importance of supervisors having well-developed interpersonal skills, especially the ability to listen actively. The following response describes one respondent's relationship with her supervisor:

> Wonderful – I feel safe and secure. I trust her implicitly. I respect her credibility to supervise me knowing she'll have insight and understanding of the incidents I bring.

What supervisees liked most about clinical supervision

All respondents gave examples of what they liked most about clinical supervision. The majority referred to the opportunities it offered, over half welcoming the opportunity to discuss practice and reflect on particular clinical incidents.

Increased intensity of workload and changing shift patterns, for example the loss of the afternoon shift overlap, may mean that, outside clinical supervision, nurses get little chance to talk with colleagues about specific work issues. In addition, minimal staffing levels have resulted in nurses taking fewer or shorter meal breaks, often in isolation, which limits opportunities for talking to trusted colleagues about incidents and feelings. Social networks used by nurses have largely disappeared as more nurses now live in private accommodation away from the hospital. Domestic responsibilities, often as a family wage earner, may also leave nurses little time for discussing the feelings that arise through work. Against this background, it is perhaps not surprising that supervisees viewed clinical supervision as:

> An opportunity to discuss things that are important to me.
>
> Time to talk knowing that someone else understands how I feel.

Nurses saw clinical supervision as a way of 'downloading' the effects of work. Many respondents used the term 'Time for me' or described clinical supervision as a chance to escape from the pressures of work in order to think more constructively.

What supervisees liked least about clinical supervision

Just over half of respondents answered this question. Some found it difficult to find time, and there was some guilt expressed about leaving the ward and busy colleagues. Although the activity evaluation suggests that most clinical supervision activity took place during duty time, there was nevertheless some concern that clinical supervision occasionally took place outside duty time. Interruptions during clinical supervision were a source of frustration, and a small number of respondents said that clinical supervision felt a bit awkward or uncomfortable until one got used to it.

Self-reported changes in attitude

Respondents were asked to say whether or not their attitude
to their work had changed as a result of clinical supervision,
and, if it had, to give an example. The two themes generated
in response to this question concerned nurses' attitudes towards
external factors, such as colleagues and work situations, and
towards themselves. A number of respondents gave examples
of changing attitudes to colleagues or said that they had become
more reflective about events occurring at work:

> I am much more willing to listen to other people's opinions. I have
> become aware of the benefits of clinical supervision as a tool for
> defusing stressful situations, particularly for less experienced nurses.

> I am able to see events from more than one perspective. It gives
> me a better understanding of the episode.

Some nurses felt more confident or had a more positive attitude as a result of receiving clinical supervision:

> Sometimes I have difficulties trying to get something positive out
> of a difficult experience. However, with the ability and confidence
> to use guided reflection I have been able to turn my dissatisfying
> incidents to move forward in a constructive useful way.

Nurses also reported changing attitudes to themselves as a
result of receiving clinical supervision. They were less likely to
'hold on to things' or blame themselves when things went wrong:

> I feel I can now discuss some worrying aspect of nursing, explore
> it and then let it go. Perhaps before I would be hanging on to a
> situation too long without coming to some form of solution. I would
> have felt more isolated in that particular worry.

> I reflect on my practice longer and in more depth at the time of
> the event and don't feel so guilty if I don't know all the right answers.

Those involved in introducing clinical supervision were
particularly encouraged to hear that nurses could develop
more positive attitudes about themselves and their work by
engaging in clinical supervision. Such attitudes are fundamental
in helping nurses to value and articulate the contribution they
make to patient care.

Self-reported changes to practice

Over two-thirds of respondents cited a wide range of examples of changes made to practice as a result of clinical supervision, as could be expected from the number of clinical settings represented. These included reviewing patient handover, the use of various assessment tools, serving meals, the use of patients' first names and meeting patients' spiritual needs, to mention but a few. As well as examples of changes to nursing practice, respondents also gave examples of changes to approaches to work, several of which involved interpersonal relationships, especially with medical colleagues.

Self-reported changes in knowledge

Just under half the respondents gave examples of how their knowledge had changed as a result of clinical supervision, although some of the responses were rather unspecific. Interestingly, more than one respondent mentioned increased knowledge related to the management of aggression and communication.

Reflections on the evaluation programme

At the end of this evaluation exercise, we gained the impression that there was enthusiasm and commitment to clinical supervision within the Trust despite constraining factors related to lack of time and other resources. Nurses were beginning to value clinical supervision as an effective professional and personal development strategy while offering the potential for improving standards of patient care. In addition, the reduction in sickness absence, the results of the Maslach inventory and the responses to the semistructured questionnaires all suggest that clinical supervision could provide nurses with a useful defence strategy for dealing with the effects of emotional labour.

At this early stage of implementing clinical supervision, there was still much to learn and discover, and many difficulties to overcome. Fortunately, the enthusiasm and commitment of our colleagues, pioneering clinical supervision in the Trust, kept us positive and alive to its benefits. The practice development team coined a phrase for clinical supervision:

time to reflect, time to think, time to learn.

Now it was time to look to the future, our vision being to ensure that every nurse employed in the Trust could, if they so wished, have *1 hour a month* of clinical supervision.

Management support

With the results of the evaluation study under her belt, the project leader sought the views and support of the Chief Executive on the full implementation of clinical supervision on a voluntary basis. She decided to go straight for the heart! How do you demonstrate that you value your staff? – clinical supervision is a way to do so. While costs must be considered, to cost the programme was incredibly convoluted, with, for example, educational/training budgets, project development monies attracted into the Trust and recruitment and retention strategies to be taken into account. The bottom line, the project leader decided, was 'Are the nurses each worth one hour a month?' While not a strictly accurate equation in view of the several hours of supervisors' time, this was nonetheless overridden by the fact that many staff would not opt in to have an hour of supervision. The Chief Executive agreed that it could not be otherwise – his staff were, of course, worth one hour a month. What was perhaps to become apparent was that staff do not necessarily value themselves that much and sometimes miss sessions, or do not enter into the programme because of 'lack of time' due to constantly increased clinical activities. Once the Chief Executive's approval had been obtained, a meeting was held with the clinical service unit managers, all of whom signed up in support. Clinical supervision was also written into the nursing strategy as an ongoing programme for implementation.

Views of some participants

Interviews were arranged between the second author, who had no formal association with the Trust, three supervisees and two supervisors. The aim of these meetings was to identify why clinical supervision had interested these professionals and what benefits they considered had resulted from the process. In common with many clinical staff, one of the supervisees had not had any previous experience of clinical supervision, although she had been using an informal mechanism for some time, which, she realised, could be maximised through clinical supervision. As with other staff interviewed, she had not been able to get to the 'think tank' but followed up the discussions that arose from it and asked to opt in. This young sister felt strongly that it should be the right of every nurse, although, she added, some had an odd view of it and the 'name needs changing'. A senior staff nurse said:

> A lot of people thought they knew all about it, but changed their mind at the end of the introductory study day, the term had misled them.

One nurse, who had been to the 'think tank', remembers sitting at the meeting thinking that it would be good for her managerially. At first, she saw clinical supervision as an albeit self-inflicted infringement – a commitment to which she had to stick – but now, as she says:

> I felt I could get away from my ward and talk to someone in confidence, someone who understands my problems. You go in, you do the work, you take an awful lot of work home with you – I don't think you should have to do that. You can't keep your motivation going all by yourself, especially when wards close and morale is low. Clinical supervision gives you that boost.

All participants, whether supervisors or supervisees, felt that clinical supervision was something into which you grew, that it was 'counselling' in a professional way, about individuals and their work. This focus on counselling is not uncommon; it is the view of some nurses that the supportive element of clinical supervision is its major function. However, other interviewees spoke of the confidence that they had developed: confidence to challenge routine practices, and to challenge others when unhappy with decisions about patients' care. One said:

> I'm more confident now, I feel I'm doing a good job, doing it well, and can reflect on what I'm doing.

Another stated:

> I think it's brilliant – it's helped me to grow. There have been so many changes in this Trust, about nurses' roles, about the combination of clinical care and management responsibilities. Supervisors provide a sounding board. They don't have all the answers but it makes you brave enough to think about it. You develop the ability to draw on experience.

Another supervisee recalled an attempt to develop an informal support group prior to the introduction of clinical supervision, but, for whatever reason, the dynamics did not work:

> I suppose what we were crying out for was clinical supervision, but we didn't know about it then!

The role of the nurse specialist can be a lonely one, even in an acute and very busy Trust, and while clinical professional support may be in abundance, there are often issues that are inappropriate to discuss with general colleagues. One nurse spoke of her first session as a supervisee being taken up with staff dynamics:

> I didn't get the answer, but it got me to think through what I'd have to do, and had half thought out. Next time anything similar comes up I'll draw from that.

Some supervisees wrote down critical incidents as well as their feelings about them, while others kept notes only of feelings, avoiding recording specific identifiable incidents, although many of the specific data would be collected through the Trust audit system. None of the participants considered that group supervision would be as useful as one-to-one supervision and saw setting the agenda for a session as very flexible. Several spoke of having a written incident to discuss, which 'hit the bin' when they walked in as a more pressing matter overwhelmed them. The intent is always to be quite structured, and supervisors were trained to accommodate instant needs without losing the agreed format of the Proctor (1992) model. One such session was described:

> I walked in deciding to talk about one thing, but when my supervisor said How are you? I just burst into tears. I wasn't coping. The whole session was about how I wasn't coping, and we had an extra session to make sure I was OK. If I hadn't had clinical supervision I don't know how I would have got it together. It's not that I don't have time to touch points with other individuals, but the safety of clinical supervision was what I really needed.

One of the supervisors had kept a reflective diary and had participated in group sessions as a student but once qualified did not see anywhere for such valuable practices to 'fit' until clinical supervision was discussed at the Trust. All of the supervisors enjoyed the training course at the university and considered it to be beneficial. Approximately every 3 months, the individuals concerned review their sessions and, if necessary, alter their format, while still keeping within the guidelines. When asked if she would be offended if, after some time, supervisees felt that they needed a different supervisor, the supervisor's response reflected the expertise and caring central to effective clinical supervision:

> I think that this is what I should be striving for. To develop my supervisees' potential which must surely mean that at some point they need more than I can give them and they should move on.

All the supervisees interviewed hoped to become supervisors and were either waiting to go on the next course or were waiting for staff levels to improve. As one nurse pointed out:

> I want to be a supervisor; I've done the course but I know that I can't be depended on just now. When staff vacancies are filled I shall go onto the directory. You can't let people down, you must be there for them.

Conclusion

We have described in detail how one acute Trust began the journey on the road to effective clinical supervision. With sound management support and the ability to negotiate our own timetable, staff were gradually brought on board, and now the main author's work is cut out to accommodate the demand. Crucial to the success to date has been the commitment and enthusiasm of the staff in the practice development unit; the importance of having an identified lead person on the subject cannot be overestimated as, with the best will in the world, people's priorities will change with conflicting agendas.

The analogy has been made that supervisors are a bit like personal trainers. They focus on the individual practitioner's goals, they help with motivation, help to stretch that little bit further, but always with the individual's own fitness and well-being in mind. While this Trust does not presume to have got clinical supervision totally right, it has no doubt that its gradual and carefully planned implementation is creating a beneficial culture to support staff in providing the quality skill and expertise that the Trust holds dear and is committed to.

References

Butterworth, T., Bishop, V. and Carson, J. 1996 First steps to evaluating clinical supervision in nursing and health visiting. Part 1: Theory, policy and practice development. A review. *Journal of Clinical Nursing* 5: 127–32.

Butterworth, T., Carson, J., White, E., Jeacock, J., Clements, A. and Bishop, V. 1997 *It Is Good to Talk. An Evaluation of Clinical Supervision and Mentorship in England and Scotland.* Manchester: University of Manchester School of Nursing and Midwifery.

Clothier, C., MacDonald, C.A. and Shaw, D.A. 1994 *The Allitt Inquiry.* London: HMSO.

Department of Health 1993 *A Vision for the Future: The Nursing, Midwifery and Health Visiting Contribution to Health and Health Care.* London: HMSO.

Hawkins, P. and Shohet, R. 1992 *Supervision in the Helping Professions.* Milton Keynes: Open University Press.

James, N. 1992 Care = organisation + physical labour = emotional labour. *Sociology of Health and Illness* 14(4): 489–509.

Marshall, M. 1994 *Controversies in Health Care Policies: Challenges to Practice.* London: BMJ Publishing Group.

Maslach, C. and Jackson, S.E. 1981 The measurement of experienced burnout. *Journal of Occupational Behaviour* 2: 99–113.

Proctor, B. 1991 On being a trainer and supervision for counselling in action. In: Hawkins, P. and Shohet, R. *Supervision in the Helping Professions*. Milton Keynes: Open University Press.

Royal College of Nursing 1995 *Clinical Supervision. Professional Update*. **3**(5).

Smith, P. 1992 *The Emotional Labour of Nursing*. Basingstoke: Macmillan.

UKCC (United Kingsom Central Council for Nursing, Midwifery and Health Visiting) 1996 *Initial Position Statement on Clinical Supervision for Nursing and Health Visiting*. London: UKCC.

6

The Development of Guidelines on Clinical Supervision in Clinical Practice Settings

Nigel Northcott

This chapter is based upon the experiences of introducing clinical supervision onto an acute medical ward, which was one of the DoH/King's Fund-supported Nursing Development Units (NDUs). The contextual issues that led to this project being part of the NDU are explored, along with the understanding of clinical supervision that framed the approach used. The scheme of clinical supervision that was agreed upon is identified, along with guidelines on good practice for clinical supervision that arose from the work. A number of the key questions arising from the staff and the response to these are offered as illustrations of some of the concerns and uncertainties that clinical supervision can generate for nurses. The chapter includes limited evaluation of the experiences on the NDU and offers the profession a case study from which to draw conclusions to inform endeavours to introduce clinical supervision elsewhere.

Introduction

In the spring of 1992, two events occurred that led to the creation of the guidelines on the use of clinical supervision, that conclude this chapter. The first was my decision to register to work towards a PhD and the second was my appointment as the clinical leader of a DoH/King's Fund-sponsored NDU, ward 7E, an acute medical ward at the John Radcliffe Hospital in Oxford. These two events allowed me to explore a number of contemporary issues that affected nurses and nursing, including the emerging idea of clinical supervision (Butterworth and Faugier, 1992). The topic of my doctoral research (North-cott, 1996a) was appraisal and professional fulfilment for nurses, arising in part from the interest and concerns I had about the support strategies available to nurses.

The central pillar of an NDU is the empowerment of patients by the empowerment of nurses, with the development of practice being one of the explicit features. These expectations, along with the commitment to share what we learnt with the profession at large (Garbett, 1992), were likely to increase the demands upon the nurses on the ward. In 1996, Scholes confirmed that additional pressure exists for nurses on an NDU. To help ameliorate that pressure on ward 7E, the use of clinical supervision was identified as a component of the ward culture (Northcott 1994, 1996b) that could help to provide the necessary support for nurses. This chapter concludes with a set of guidelines on clinical supervision inspired by my experience as the clinical leader of ward 7E over a 3-year period. The chapter explains how these guidelines were created and, using the experience of the nurses on the NDU, answers a number of the questions about clinical supervision that developed in action.

It is essential at the outset to appreciate the textuality of this experience with clinical supervision. Usher and Edwards (1994) offer a framework for interrogating textuality that is useful to consider before proceeding:

- *Con-text* – the things that were going on at the time. This includes the changes to health care management, the new status as an NDU, the appointment of a new clinical leader and project workers, the imperative to explore practice and the expectation to contribute broadly to the development of nursing.
- *Pre-text* – what preceded the introduction, including the ward culture and working patterns, and historical issues.
- *Sub-text* – what underpins the situation, such as the professional issues, hidden agendas and power relationships.

The realisation of contextual significance confirms the need to apply clinical supervision to *each* clinical setting and recognise that no one model is universally applicable even within the microculture of one hospital or clinical unit. Indeed, I would go so far as to suggest that the exact approach used should be unique to each individual nurse, within locally agreed ground rules and models. However, the experiences of others, along with their guidelines, or for example a position statement, such as that from the UKCC (1996), can help to facilitate the emergence of clinical supervision in any setting.

Initially, the timing of my appointment to ward 7E and the commencement of work towards my PhD seemed unfortunate in terms of the demands they created. However, the common ground between them made it a highly attractive opportunity that proved fruitful in many ways. Developing knowledge and awareness of performance management in my doctoral research, and leading a team of nurses to be innovative and creative, proved to have much in common. The importance of ensuring the appropriate level of support (an essential aspect of performance management) led us in the spring of 1994 to clinical supervision. This chapter describes the contextuality and details of the approach to clinical supervision that arose on ward 7E and concludes with a set of guidelines that I continue to use in my current work.

Personal context and background

In 1992, I was working in the Oxfordshire Clinical Education and Practice Team (OXCEPT) as a facilitator and the team leader. The role was based around the use of education as a means to effect change, enhance practice, improve effectiveness and develop services and individuals. OXCEPT is both reactive to the needs of nurses (latterly all health care staff) and proactive to try to predict the activities that contemporary practice would need. The team runs educational events, provides role-based development and facilitation for individuals and groups, which since 1994 has included workshops on clinical supervision. The guidelines on clinical supervision concluding this chapter that developed from the work on ward 7E continue to be used in this work in OXCEPT.

As a result of my facilitator's role in OXCEPT, I was acutely aware that increasing demands upon all nurses arose from the expectations of the 1990s health industry and from a growing number of professional initiatives. The project by the UKCC (Professional Practice and Education Project; UKCC, 1990), the document Scope of Professional Practice (UKCC, 1992a) and unprecedented educational demands created pressures for the whole profession. I set out in my doctoral research to explore the value and impact of appraisal for nurses as one means to provide support and was keenly aware that a number of strategies existed to assist nurses to meet challenges. Early in my thesis, I acknowledge the work of Daloz (1987, p. 214), who, in exploring the role of mentorship to promote effective education, creates a grid that represents the relationship between support and challenge. I have modified the grid as in Figure 6.1.

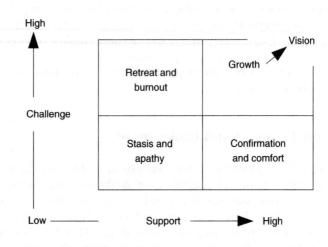

Figure 6.1   The challenge and support dimensions and their interactive results (Northcott, 1996a; after Daloz, 1987)

I was acutely aware that the dimensions of challenge and support both had to operate as 'high' if the expectations and aspirations of nurses and nursing were to be met satisfactorily. I suspected that the low-challenge dimension was unlikely to exist organisationally, as the NHS in the 1990s strove to be more effective and efficient, but such a situation might exist for individuals. The high-challenge scenario that produces 'burnout' is well documented with regard to nurses (Maslach, 1982; Whitehead, 1989). Marcellison *et al.* (1988) report that strong social support could assist workers to cope with 'job stressors'. The great pressure that carers such as nurses experience is well documented (Cooper, 1988; Wolfgang, 1988) and Hingly and Harris (1986) compound this concern by asserting that the nursing profession at times neglects support for nurses, seeing it as a concern of the individual.

As an educationalist, I was particularly aware of the impact upon individuals of trying to effect change that is explored in the work of Jack Mezirow on 'perspective transformation' (Mezirow, 1981). This process of creating disorientation, of exploration and eventual reintegration, is considered as 'macro-reflection' of a type that strives to explore practice within the context. This approach sees education as a process of change that has an emotional tariff as well as influencing intellect and, hopefully, practice. In April 1992, when I was appointed as the part-time clinical leader of ward 7E, I was aware that the NDU status would add to the change and challenges (perspective transformation[s]) that the nurses on the ward would be exposed to and experience. I was particularly sensitive to the importance of a facilitator (teacher) to help manage the disequilibrium. Brookfield (1987) identifies the value of a 'helper' to facilitate the learning process, and I anticipated this need for the nurses on ward 7E as they undertook the additional responsibilities of being an NDU. I was aware that I would be unable to provide this 'help' alone and therefore sought a means by which I could share the responsibility that reflected the management ethos and culture on the ward.

The changing work of nurses

The work of nurses had, by the early 1990s, experienced major organisational change as traditional autonomy for decision-making once invested in the ward sister (Ersser and Tutton, 1991) had been devolved to individual practitioners within the philosophy and practice of primary nursing (Vaughan, 1989). Indeed, in part, I was attracted to the post on ward 7E because of this, and I would rely upon it, as I was appointed part time on secondment from my role in OXCEPT. The highly developed practice of primary nursing on ward 7E was a legacy I gratefully inherited for both professional and personal reasons. The dynamic nursing workforce, who were used to individual responsibility and change, were ready to accept the challenges of an NDU. Primary nursing was well established in an organisational framework of team nursing on the ward, and I was able to rely upon a devolved management style that challenged the nurses to bring about development. I recognised that within this context, as the clinical leader, I had a particular remit to ensure that there were support strategies in place consistent with the level of challenge of an NDU. This would leave the nurses to manage the nursing, and my role as managing them.

The approach that I took to this managerial role was based upon subsidiarity: 'stealing other people's responsibilities is wrong' (Handy, 1994). The delegation of the management of care to the nurses within the framework of primary nursing required an approach to leadership that was 'there for them' when it was needed but not controlling or directing. My role was to sustain the right culture, ensure that a suitable psychological contract existed and reinforce the principles of stewardship. Block (1993) describes stewardship as 'accountability *without* control or compliance, but *with* support and nurturing'. I aspired to provide leadership that would, as Bennis and Nanus (1985) suggest, translate 'intention into reality'. To ensure success, I considered three management concepts to be central to the aspirations of an NDU and in particular to the approach to nursing care management that operated on the ward.

Culture, psychological contracts and stewardship

These three management concepts informed the running of the NDU and significantly facilitated the introduction of clinical supervision as a developmental strategy to support individual accountability.

I would like to suggest that autocracy, macho management and management by directive that seeks to control staff are unlikely either to need or to value clinical supervision. It is also unlikely that any clinical area operating thus would aspire to develop practice or its staff. I make no claim that the absence of clinical supervision negates quality care, or that an auto-cratic approach to management prevents innovation. However, there does appear to be a causal link between developed prac-tice and developmental approaches to management that includes the use of clinical supervision. This in part explains the coincidental establishment of clinical supervision on a ward recognised by the DoH and King's Fund as an NDU.

The culture, or 'how things are done around here' was central to the NDU, and Rob Garbett, one of the project leaders, used the term 'family' to describe the ward nursing team (Garbett, 1993). It was a ward team of nurses that recognised conflict as part of everyday life and which worked towards solutions as a 'learning company'. The 'learning company' as promoted by Pedlar *et al.* (1991) is one in which learning, feedback, change and evaluation are all central, and these are the cardinal features of an NDU. The culture was recognised as a dynamic feature of the NDU that developed as the staff on the NDU devel-oped. Integral to the culture of the NDU was its nursing philos-ophy, which was again a dynamic feature of the ward and was subject to regular revisions to ensure its accuracy (Garbett, 1994).

The psychological contract (Northcott, 1996c) covers a range of implied and usually unstated expectations that influence performance. The contract includes mutual expectations: in exchange for the use of talents and energies, the organisation makes certain provisions for the staff. The expectation for nursing was to provide high standards of care, delivered in a manner that respected individual rights and wishes. The nurses were required to be creative, be reflective and use knowledge to underpin practice. The provision from nurse managers (the clinical leader and team leaders) of support and encourage-ment was typified by the commitment to provide clinical super-vision. Taken together, these established a psychological contract in which, in exchange for quality care, team members were nurtured.

Stewardship (Block, 1993) is a management approach that requires leaders who recognise their role as that of 'caretaker', in which being the director who controls is replaced by being a conductor who co-ordinates. Stewardship recognises that organisations have a culture persisting beyond their term of office and which sees customers as central to work. It is an approach to management that reflects empowerment and deprecates control and coercion.

The learning culture of the NDU, a psychological contract that recognised staff needs and a leadership style in which I functioned as manager of last resort all worked to value devolution and individual responsibility. The culture recognised the place of change and the pressure this might put upon the staff. Stewardship is as much about empowerment of patients by nurses as it is about empowerment of nurses by their leaders: a cardinal feature of an NDU. The culture and managerial approach were central features of the NDU and were crucial to the success of the ward in its developmental role, which in turn both necessitated and facilitated the introduction of clinical supervision. The factors that precipitated the introduction of clinical supervision on ward 7E were the continuous responsibility for admissions as one of the six acute medical wards for the city, the additional pressures of being an NDU and a culture and management style that valued the staff. The high bed occupancy, high patient dependency and high patient turnover on the ward created sufficient demands in themselves to promote the introduction of clinical supervision.

Given that there were 22 whole-time equivalent nurses on ward 7E, it was impractical for me to provide support for all the nurses by way of clinical supervision. The use of primary nursing in teams on the ward had led to the establishment of three team leaders who, along with the two project workers and clinical leader (the ward management team), provided a pool of senior colleagues. I explored various models of support (the helper role) promoted for nurses that might be appropriate to these circumstances. Brookfield (1987) identifies the role of 'helper' to facilitate learning in a broad educational sense, and the role has manifested itself in nursing and beyond as mentor, appraiser, preceptor and as clinical supervisor.

Mentor, appraiser, preceptor or clinical supervisor?

Mentor, appraiser, preceptor and clinical supervisor all recognise the need for the dual actions of challenge and support to ensure that change and growth arise. Deciding which of these would accommodate the needs of the staff on ward 7E was the subject of much debate among the ward staff. 'Mentor' was the term used for the undergraduate nurse education programme in Oxfordshire and was therefore recognised by the staff. However, the role included formal assessment of performance, which was not a feature required for supporting qualified nurses. 'Preceptor' was identified by the UKCC as 'good practice' (UKCC, 1990) and was seen particularly as a strategy to assist newly appointed and newly qualified staff but not to provide longitudinal support to trained nurses. I was so uncertain about the status and operation of appraisal for nurses that I was embarking upon an extended piece of research into it. At the time, the hospital had no clear guidelines on appraisal, and the initial explorations for my research revealed apathy and dissatisfaction with it. The nurses on the NDU supported these views on appraisal, and few of them had recent or favourable attitudes to report. In the light of these circumstances, I felt that the need for support might best be met from a 'new' approach – clinical supervision.

I explored the literature on clinical supervision available in the early 1990s, such as Butterworth and Faugier (1992) and Hawkins and Shohet (1989). I decided that an interaction between a supervisor and a supervisee, which aims to assist the latter to develop and become more effective, was an ideal strategy for ward 7E. The recognition that clinical supervision could enhance the individual and the organisation by using an agenda created by the supervisee would enhance any clinical area and reflect the aspirations and intentions of the NDU.

The three aims for clinical supervision that Veronica Bishop promoted in 1994 – to safeguard standards, to develop professional expertise and to deliver quality care – all reflect the aspirations of an NDU. The impact of clinical supervision to assist the individual to conceptualise practice, to advance a philosophy of that practice and to explore issues of concern would provide the support that I speculated was needed. The demands of change that were inherent in an NDU necessitated support that was comprehensive and centred on the individual. The idea that clinical supervision was a formal opportunity (a legitimate workplace activity) to informally (in a nurturing and developmental culture) explore work suggested that it would provide the support required.

First steps towards clinical supervision – annual performance review and learning contracts

The framework for clinical supervision that we eventually used on ward 7E arose from experimenting with appraisal (annual review and planning), learning contracts, and the identified need for support (mentorship or similar). Early in 1993, I raised with the management team on the ward my concerns about ensuring that appropriate support existed for the nurses in the absence of a functioning appraisal scheme. I was reluctant to introduce a new appraisal scheme part way through my own research but felt that something was needed. We recognised that learning contracts had become an established feature on the ward, given that most of the registered nurses acted as 'mentors' to the undergraduate nurses. The method of assessing competence in clinical placements for our student nurse colleagues was by means of a learning contract. However, in order that we might create appropriate learning contracts, we first needed some means to identify the learning needs with each individual registered nurse.

Annual performance review/evaluation

The NDU had identified goals and clinical projects as part of its status, and the nurses were conversant with broader professional aspirations. The requirement was for a means to assist them in summarising their current performance, as a benchmark from which to establish their development needs. Unlike the conventional approach used in appraisal schemes, such as IPR (NHSTA, 1986), of a boss-led evaluation, we felt that a broader base was required. It was for this reason that the annual performance review form had a number of sections as shown in Box 6.1.

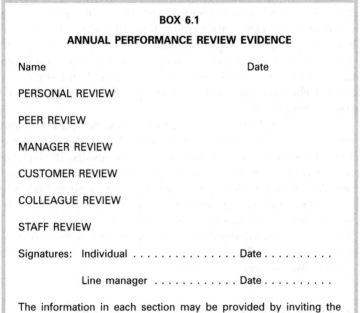

BOX 6.1

ANNUAL PERFORMANCE REVIEW EVIDENCE

Name   Date

PERSONAL REVIEW

PEER REVIEW

MANAGER REVIEW

CUSTOMER REVIEW

COLLEAGUE REVIEW

STAFF REVIEW

Signatures: Individual . . . . Date . . . .

                 Line manager . . . . Date . . . .

The information in each section may be provided by inviting the appropriate person to write directly onto the review, or by the individual completing a summary. The review may be used directly or indirectly to complete a departmental annual review. The customer review might be third party information, spontaneous feedback or indeed solicited evaluation. The staff review section should only be completed by staff with line management responsibility.

The categories used on the review form reflect the extent of the nurses' role and the value of feedback from a number of sources. The responsibility for collating the data and keeping the sheet rested with the individual nurse. This assessment, even without formally filling it in, enabled the nurse, along with a senior colleague, to complete appropriate learning contracts, called 'personal development contracts'.

Personal development contracts

The exact model of each contract varied according to the individual nurse and the senior colleague with whom they worked. Box 6.2 gives an example of such a contract, set out on one side of A4 paper to keep it concise. This was to accommodate staff concerns that both the undergraduates' and their own learning contracts on post-registration modules had been overly large and unwieldy.

The successful use of the annual reviews and learning contracts was limited in the first year, although a number of nurses used both approaches with notable results. In part, the introduction of these was overtaken by interest and enthusiasm for clinical supervision. A memo sent to all staff in May 1994, following the agreement of the team leaders to offer clinical supervision, was greeted enthusiastically by the nurses. The memo acknowledged the start made with annual reviews and learning contracts, and invited nurses to accommodate these within clinical supervision.

Model of clinical supervision on ward 7E

The approach to clinical supervision that was to be considered was circulated to all the nurses and is presented in Box 6.3. The approach was intended to be personalised by each nurse and was presented as guidelines to allow for this interpretation, with only one universal standard.

BOX 6.2

PERSONAL DEVELOPMENT CONTRACT

Date. . . . . Contract number . . . .

Name   i . . . .

Helper   ii . . . .

Line Manager   iii. . . . .

IDENTIFIED NEED/GOAL (**S**pecific, **T**imely, **A**chievable and **R**ealistic).

OUTCOMES TO MEET NEED

RESOURCES NEEDED

TIMETABLE

PROGRESS, EVALUATION and REVIEWS

Agreement signatures   i . . . .

                               ii . . . .

                               iii. . . . .

Date . . . .

Achievement signatures   i . . . .

                               ii . . . .

                               iii. . . . .

Date . . . .

Note. This sample of a learning contract recognises that the helper(s) may be different from the line manager, and that agreement includes the provision of support by the helper(s) and manager.

BOX 6.3

THE WARD 7E/NDU APPROACH TO CLINICAL SUPERVISION IN 1994

7E/NDU Professional Supervision/Appraisal

Introduction
The scheme of Professional Supervision/Appraisal set out here reflects current thinking on performance management. The scheme is designed to incorporate mentorship, preceptorship appraisal and supervision. Individuals are encouraged to modify the practice to meet individual needs. There is however one standard:

Supervision sessions of at least 30 minutes should be held at least every 8 weeks for all staff during work time.

In the early stages meetings may need to be more frequent and of longer duration.

The Scheme
Philosophy: The underlying principle that should guide the activity is *development* and *growth*. Professional staff work to codes of conduct that set out their responsibility and this scheme acknowledges the integrity of this principle.

Who: The activity should accommodate the needs of the *individual* and of their *role*. For this reason an up-to-date job description and philosophy of the ward are essential to guide the activity. It should be recognised that performance is influenced by team colleagues and other professionals that are worked with.

Organisational culture: Like the overall philosophy of the ward, the culture within which supervision/appraisal occurs is *development*, with the ward striving to be a *learning company*.

Focus: The focus of the supervision/appraisal is by the joint approaches of challenge and support. To optimise performance, high challenge and high support are essential. Too little challenge or too little support will not obtain the best performance, and absence of them both will result in the least development of potential.

Purposes: The use of supervision/appraisal has a number of benefits both to the individual and to the organisation. These include enhancing performance and increasing dialogue between staff, and ensuring a professional performance is achieved. It is *not* envisaged that that activity will be used to influence pay or promotion nor as a disciplinary action.   *cont'd*

BOX 6.3 (cont'd)

Approach: Two strategies are commended to the staff: professional supervision and progress review. The details of the approaches are as follows:

Professional supervision, with three purposes:

- support (restorative element) to assist in managing the existing workload and to help with the pressure of extending skills into other areas.
- education (formative element) to provide information, networks and ideas to underpin and extend practice.
- management (normative element) to help practitioners discharge their accountability as a professional.

One of the core activities of professional supervision should be reflective practice, an activity designed to ensure experiences are used for learning. The supervisor fulfils the 'helper' role, to support and listen to enable the individual to make sense of an experience. There are three stages to this process:

- What happened?
- How did it make me feel ? (How might colleagues and patients feel?)
- How should I act in the future as a result?

Keeping a private diary with reflective notes will help you keep track of events that shape your professional development. These notes could be held within your personal portfolio/profile and, if appropriate, shared at supervision.

Progress review: an annual meeting of at least an hour provided to establish the following cycle.

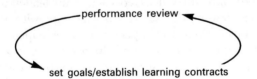

The review should include the production of half a side of A4 as a summary of the year for the individual which could be included in the ward annual review. The performance review should set goals/learning contracts for the following year. It is envisaged that learning contracts could be set at any time during the year, but should be restricted to five active ones at any time.   *cont'd*

BOX 6.3 (cont'd)

Who: The *supervisor* is most likely to be your team leader, but it is suggested that no more than six people should be supervised by the same person.

Footnote These are guidelines and it is anticipated that local variations may be desirable and, if mutually agreed, are fully acceptable.

These guidelines were distributed to all the staff, along with a short reference list. Copies of relevant articles and sections from key texts were made available to the nurses in the ward communication folder. To facilitate the introduction, a cascade to promote the activity was used rather than the provision of formal educational or training sessions. The nurses on the NDU were conversant with the use of learning contracts, performance evaluation and the use of reflection. The culture of the ward was one that placed importance upon justifying practice and professional accountability, and, most significantly, operated as a 'learning company'. I decided that my providing supervision for the team leaders and project workers would facilitate them to offer the same for their team members to help us explore the whole process 'in action'. This approach to introducing a new idea reflects the central philosophy of the nurses' *Code of Conduct* (UKCC, 1992b), nurses being expected to act within their own limitations of expertise and seek support if they encountered difficulties. I asked each team leader to give me a brief overview of the supervisory activity with their team members during their own supervision. This helped me to evaluate their progress and provided them with an opportunity to obtain support and clarify issues. The success of introducing clinical supervision in this manner was soon evident as slots of time began to be identified on the duty roster indicating that supervision sessions were planned.

In the years that have followed this introduction, I have continued to explore clinical supervision for nurses and have regularly modified the original guidelines. This dynamic approach is manifest in the 'latest' guidelines that conclude this chapter. These arose from the NDU experience and have been created to assist nurses in all clinical settings, including those with a culture unlike the NDU. However, I must acknowledge that the early success we experienced on ward 7E with clinical supervision was strongly supported by the ward culture, and I must caution against attempts to *impose* clinical supervision as a top-down edict, especially if the culture is not conducive to change and development. Clinical supervision is a practice that can help to develop staff performance as part of a culture and context in which challenge and support are seen as closely interrelated. It may therefore be necessary for clear leadership to introduce the concept and to promote clinical supervision by helping to create a draft(s) and by accommodating the views of the staff. This approach, as used on the NDU, focuses on strong leadership in conjunction with consultation and ensures that clinical supervision becomes established by mutual consent and enthusiasm.

Evaluation of the approach used on ward 7E

A year after introducing the supervision scheme, the brief comment shown in Box 6.4 was published in the NDU annual report for 1994–95 from one of the team leaders.

This evaluation echoes the importance of the relationship that facilitated clinical supervision on ward 7E, as well as indicating the benefit the nurses derived from it. However, it would not indicate the full picture to conclude on this high note as, in the early weeks, a number of questions were asked by the nurses. These were essential to fine tuning the approach as they represented the consumers' perspective. If as an NDU, we were indeed to empower staff, the scheme of supervision had to be developed to ensure this was possible. It was also likely that ownership of the scheme would enhance the uptake.

The questions asked were in both a written and an oral format. Nurses on occasions directly challenged me or other members of the ward management team or used the ward communication folder to ask for clarification. These questions and the solutions that were offered complemented the first year of development of clinical supervision on the NDU and have informed the guidelines.

BOX 6.4

**EVALUATION OF CLINICAL SUPERVISION ON
WARD 7E/NDU BY A TEAM LEADER**

The model of supervision that developed on ward 7E aimed to give support to all staff and encourage personal and professional development. Reflective practice is encouraged, both on a one-to-one basis with the supervisor and latterly in groups, with the main aim of improving patient care. The use of learning contracts directs individuals' work towards personal objectives, with support coming from their supervisor. Supervisory sessions occur at least every 8 weeks, for 30 minutes, and are tailored to individual needs. Essential to success has been the commitment of both nurses to the process and, in particular, to meeting regularly. I have found the relationship with my supervisor essential to the process. The feedback from her with regard to patients' satisfaction, her passing on peers' evaluation of my practice and her comments have all helped my confidence to grow. Prior to working on ward 7E I had not worked on an acute ward for 2 years, and supervision was a vital element in supporting me to develop. Since coming to ward 7E, I have been encouraged to take responsibility for my own development and to make my own career goals, which, along with the supervision, has allowed me to develop my career.

Questions and answers about clinical supervision from ward 7E/NDU

'What if I don't want supervision?'

You are under no obligation to enter into clinical supervision. It is optional for all staff and, as the agenda should arise from you, there would be no point forcing you to take part. The ward management team feels that the demands and challenges of a busy ward, let alone an NDU, warrant a specific support strategy for the staff. We have chosen to offer this approach to all the nurses to complement mentorship and preceptorship. We realise that some of the nurses on ward 7E are using mentors of their own choice both within the ward and outside, and wish to encourage this. We have chosen to offer clinical supervision as we think it is more comprehensive and provides a natural follow-on from preceptorship. All nurses newly appointed to ward 7E will continue to be asked to work as supernumerary in their first week and have a named peer allocated to assist their orientation to the ward.

Comment

There was initially a small degree of disinterest and reluctance from a few of the nurses. However, the feedback from their peers in time reassured them, and within 3 months all the nurses were engaged in the scheme. This answer also stimulated further questions about the exact nature of the different approaches to support. A side of A4 notes on mentorship, preceptorship and clinical supervision was placed into the ward communication folder to set out the differences and offer an extensive reading list. However, as the next question shows, this was still not sufficient.

'What is the difference between clinical supervision, professional supervision and supervision?'

The active use of supervision for nurses in acute settings is fairly new, although it is well established for psychiatric nurses and in professions such as social work and the probation service. Supervision has always existed as one of the functions of management. This type of supervision (management supervision) is the continuous process of monitoring the practice of all staff to safeguard patients and is the responsibility of your immediate line manager (team leader) and senior colleagues. It operates according to the hospital disciplinary procedure and is seldom used or indeed needed. Management supervision will continue as before on ward 7E, as on all wards, to ensure safe practice.

Supervision, or 'super-vision', focuses upon providing support and challenge to develop *all* the nurses, and there is debate about the right term for this process, especially as there is the risk of confusion with 'management supervision'. This is the reason why terms such as 'clinical' and 'professional' are used, and there are even suggestions that an altogether new term is needed. We have chosen to use 'clinical' as the first word, to distinguish between management supervision and because the aim is to focus upon developing *clinical* practice.

'Who will see the records of our supervision?'

Individual nurses will be responsible for their own records and can decide whom to share them with. Supervisors should keep track of the 'events' and of issues they need to follow up but do not need to keep a comprehensive record of the content of the supervision. It is suggested that your records should be kept within your professional profile as they will constitute ideal evidence of development for the UKCC with regard to PREP (UKCC, 1990).

'Why can't I choose my supervisor?'

You can, with the proviso that the clinical leader agrees with your choice. This is to ensure that you choose a colleague who is able to provide the appropriate support. If you wish to have supervision from a colleague other than your team leader please ask them or the clinical leader, to help you identify an alternative.

Comment

Three of the nurses asked for supervision from a colleague other than their team leader. One D grade nurse was permitted to use an E grade colleague in her own team who was considered to have the necessary expertise and who felt competent. However, two nurses who asked if they could supervise each other were advised against this and invited to reconsider their choice. This was not to say that peer supervision was not seen to be an appropriate model but that, with their limited professional experience, I was fearful they would not be fully supportive, and there was a risk of the relationship becoming 'consensus collusion'. This can arise if staff fail to realise that clinical supervision, as a developmental activity, requires challenge as well as support. The two nurses in question on the NDU wanted to meet together over a glass of wine to 'chat about work away from work'. They agreed that this could become heavy on support and lacking in sufficient challenge, and subsequently chose new supervisors.

'Why is management a feature of the model if as you suggest this is clinical and not management supervision?'

Management as used within the triangle of terms 'management', 'support' and 'education' relates to the intention that clinical supervision should help you to develop your practice from the broader perspective. This will be achieved by exploring with you professional issues, quality and, in particular, standards of practice, which are of course managerial concerns. The intention of all aspects of clinical supervision will remain developmental, your supervisor being expected to use his or her additional experience to help direct your practice.

It is not an opportunity for the supervisor to control your practice. However, if as a result of your supervision agenda, your supervisor identifies that a serious breach of practice has occurred, they must, under the requirement of the UKCC Code of Conduct, ensure that you submit yourself to the scrutiny of your colleagues or they will be obliged to report the issue to the clinical leader or to nursing management. It is anticipated that will be a very rare occurrence. If, regrettably, a serious breach of practice does occur, it is in the nurse's best interests to precipitate the enquiry by fully accepting the responsibility for any serious shortcoming.

'What should we talk about?'

The agenda within clinical supervision should arise predominantly from the supervisee, and a figure of 80 per cent of the time might be about right. The content should arise from practice and could include critical incident analysis or reflection on clinical experiences. These incidents should include occasions when you felt your practice was good as well as when you felt you could have improved. Having good practice confirmed seems to be something that nurses are not very good at. Your supervisor may also raise issues arising from your practice or from other sources that they feel you might benefit from exploring.

Comment

The supervisors were, in most cases, the nurse's team leader and therefore ideally placed to raise issues relating to the nurse's practice that would be useful agenda items. Nurses often arrived at supervision sessions with a 'list' of issues that they wished to consider; if not, asking them to recall significant recent events always created an agenda. This included ethical issues, questions about clinical activity, mentoring undergraduate nurses, vivid personal experiences and issues relating to the theory–practice interface.

'How often should we meet, for how long and where?'

The ward standard of '30 minutes every 8 weeks at work' is an advised baseline. You and your supervisor must decide on a pattern, but I suggest that you keep to at least every 8 weeks, in part to establish a pattern of meeting. It is likely that, early in the relationship, you may need to meet for longer to establish ground rules and decide how to proceed. Once a pattern has been established, you may find that you seek out your supervisor spontaneously, and for this reason your formal meetings may become shorter. I suggest you meet at work, in part to establish clinical supervision as a legitimate part of work. The NDU office is an ideal room to book for your supervision, as are the floor seminar rooms. Try to avoid the ward office as this is rarely undisturbed. You can, of course, go off the ward to anywhere that is quiet. Try to fit in sessions at the beginning or end of your shift or to take an extended lunch together.

However, if you find this difficult and you use time outside your shift, you can accumulate this into time off as hours owing.

Comment

In practice, the timing of sessions and their duration varied from time to time and nurse to nurse. Indeed, some of the formal sessions became very short as some of the supervisees took to seeking spontaneous support and exploration with their supervisor.

'Who will supervise you?'

One of the models identified in the literature is that of peer supervision, and, given the open (challenging and supportive) relationship that I have with the team leaders and project workers, I am able to obtain clinical supervision from them. However, I am not necessarily setting a precedent for peer supervision nor adopting a model that could not operate for other staff if desired.

Comment

I feel that this is a very important issue and I strongly recommend that nurses who offer supervision should also be in receipt of it. This allows them to gain personal understanding of the process and to safeguard their own skill base and well-being.

'What training will we receive to be supervised or even to be supervisors?'

The culture on ward 7E that celebrates change, exploration and a readiness to explore new ideas provides an ideal setting to 'try out' clinical supervision. This leaves me confident that we can introduce clinical supervision by a cascade from myself and the team leaders. I am confident that we have the culture to learn how to provide quality clinical supervision by doing it.

Comment

We spent several months exploring the notion of clinical supervision and decided we had to start somewhere. We anticipated that the early guidelines would require modifying in light of our experiences, and I have indeed undertaken this on several occasions. Ward 7E had an operating structure of primary nursing in teams and, as such, the team leaders were the ideal supervisors but, as reported earlier, several of the nurses stepped outside that (hierarchical) model. This approach allowed us internally to evaluate the process and modify it to reflect our experiences. I obtained direct or indirect feedback from the nurses who were providing clinical supervision on the process, and together we were able to evaluate and develop our skills. I would conclude from our experience that, in a learning culture that is supportive and inventive, clinical supervision can be established without formal training. The approach to be used should be negotiated with all the staff, with the realisation that the introduction will be a dynamic process that might take months to fine tune. However, I would also say that the imposition of a model and approach across a Trust, directorate, ward or department is likely to fail and compromises the intention of clinical supervision to help develop the practice of individual nurses.

Evaluation of the approach to clinical supervision

It had been anticipated that the NDU would run on beyond the timespan of funding from the DoH, but this did not happen. This did not affect the culture and function of the ward but did lead to the project workers and clinical leader moving on. As a result, the formal evaluation of clinical supervision that was planned for spring 1995 did not happen. I returned to OXCEPT as the full-time team leader, completed my research and continued to work on clinical supervision from an academic and educational perspective.

The work on clinical supervision set out above has been complemented by contributing to a number of workshops and conferences, and helping individual clinical nurses to explore the topic and use it in their practice. Additionally, the experience on the NDU with clinical supervision enabled me to contribute to the work undertaken by the King's Fund Centre (Kohner, 1994a). The guidelines that were published by the Centre (Kohner, 1994b) under the title *Clinical Supervision*, which I had helped to create, gave me the inspiration to use this approach. My ongoing experience with clinical supervision, both on the NDU and latterly within OXCEPT, has encouraged me to revise the guidelines I produced on the NDU on a number of occasions. I now have no idea which edition the guidelines at the end of this chapter are but can be sure they will have moved on again before you read them!

I appreciate that I stand guilty of failing formally to evaluate the effectiveness of clinical supervision on the NDU, but the change in circumstances did not permit this. However, I do feel confident to report a number of features of the NDU that I think are in part attributable to the operation of clinical supervision on the ward.

One of the cardinal features of an NDU is its ability to sustain and nurture project work that strives to explore practice. Ward 7E had two identified posts as project workers, and, during the 3 years, the contributions of these two nurses were significant. However, what was equally exciting were the clinical projects in which a large number of the ward staff were engaged which were enhanced by the support and encouragement that clinical supervision provided. Many of these projects were spawned, nurtured and cajoled into fruition in parallel to an emerging model of clinical supervision and were an unexpected and particularly exciting feature of the NDU. The clinical projects completed include a bereavement booklet, an examination of complementary therapies, shift handover auditing, wound management guidance, organisation of care audit (Adair and Murray, 1995) and exploring the views of part-time nurses (Corder, 1996).

Ward 7E also experienced three interesting features related to personnel management: a low sickness level, a high turnover and a significantly positive attitude towards part-time staff. The sickness level was lower on ward 7E than the other comparable medical wards in the hospital and was one of the lowest in the hospital. The turnover rate, however, was higher than all the comparable wards which at first glance was cause for concern. Closer scrutiny (reported in the NDU annual report of 1994–95) revealed that the destination of these staff was quite remarkable, as indicated in Box 6.5.

BOX 6.5

EXTRACT FROM WARD 7E/NDU REPORT 1994–95

During a 38-month period from January 1992 to April 1995, 35 nurses, from an establishment of 24 whole-time equivalents, resigned their position on ward 7E.

- 6 left for full or part-time education.
- 11 left for promotion to the next grade.
- 3 left for domestic reasons.
- 10 left to develop their career.
- 4 left to travel.
- 1 returned to the seconding post.

- 8 of these 35 nurses have gained further promotion since leaving ward 7E.
- 9 nurses were internally promoted to the next grade on ward 7E (these are not counted within the 35 resignations above).

In addition, 12 nurses who had worked on ward 7E since 1990 currently hold a post of grade G or above, including two lecturer practitioners, an assistant director of nursing and an editor at the *Nursing Times*. This success cannot, of course, be solely attributed to the NDU or clinical supervision, but I contest that these are important factors.

Ward 7E had a dedicated number of nurses who worked part time, and the ward was enthusiastic about using this resource. Indeed, we even recruited nurses from other medical wards who wished to go part time. This enabled good clinical nurses who, for example, wished to study, raise a family or pursue a portfolio career to remain in practice.

Finally, I would like explain the phrase 'by the formal opportunity to discuss work informally with a colleague', which is used in the second paragraph of the guidelines. This definition summarises for me what clinical supervision was about for the NDU and what it established. Nurses are now so busy that time to talk to each other has become a rare luxury. Gone are the coffee breaks together in the hospital dining room, and for too many nurses lunch is snatched in the ward office or not taken at all. The model of clinical supervision on ward 7E re-established the importance of talking in an informal setting as a formal part of ward life. It was a formal opportunity in the sense that it was acknowledged to be a vital feature of a busy ward where supporting and developing the staff were foremost in the culture. The operation of clinical supervision also appeared to produce an increase in the constructive dialogue between all staff. It encouraged reflection and exploration of practice issues with colleagues as part of the clinical supervision but also was an integral feature of ward life.

Ultimately, research projects such as the DoH-funded investigation undertaken at Manchester University by Tony Butterworth provide us with a great deal more evidence about clinical supervision. In the meantime, as an educationalist with a keen eye on the market, the continuing demand, especially from practitioners, indicates a valued product. Much of the work of a team such as OXCEPT relies upon word of mouth commendation as well as requests from staff. The demand for facilitated events on clinical supervision has shown a steady increase over the past 2 years both in Oxford and beyond, demand that I suggest speaks for itself.

Guidelines on clinical supervision

The guidelines in Box 6.6 are an update on the originals from ward 7E that were created in September 1996. They are published in full with the invitation to reproduce them as a starting point for discussions in other settings, with the proviso that the source be clearly acknowledged. They represent the work of a number of nurses from the NDU, who I trust will accept this tribute as a personal thank you. Any errors in this account I accept to be fully my responsibility.

In principle, the guidelines stand alone, but, to ensure that the message from ward 7E is unambiguous, I would like to emphasise a number of points:

- The guidelines should be used to inform local agreements, which should include where, when and who.
- Clinical supervision should focus upon the development of nursing and nurses.
- The term 'management' used in the guidelines should not be taken to imply control.
- Record-keeping should reflect the whole ethos by being supervisee held.
- Training to be supervised or to be a supervisor should be needs driven. The use of a facilitated cascade has the advantage of being introduced in a way that can fine tune the process in action and is highly recommended.
- Involvement by supervisees should be voluntary, with the onus upon facilitators to offer an attractive approach. This should include choice if not agreement about the supervisor.
- Clinical supervision should be clearly distinguished from other management functions such as midwifery supervision and management supervision.
- The process should be evaluated in some way to help monitor the impact and moderate the approach.

BOX 6.6

CLINICAL SUPERVISION – GUIDELINES FOR GOOD PRACTICE

These guidelines present a flexible approach to clinical supervision for nurses (nurses, midwives and health visitors), and are in part a response to the enthusiasm within the profession. They are intended for all grades of nurse, are designed to assist in both supervising and having supervision, and should inform local agreements on the practice.

cont'd

BOX 6.6 (cont'd)

The role of supervision is to sustain and develop clinical practice *by the formal opportunity to discuss work informally with a colleague.* Clinical supervision should focus upon supporting the development of individual nurses and not be a purely management function or a means to control practice. This is distinct from appraisal, which uses performance evaluation to set goals to help develop potential and can be operated in conjunction with clinical supervision.

The overall aims
Bishop (1994) identifies three overall aims that supervision can help nurses meet:

- a safeguard for standards of practice;
- the development of professional expertise;
- the delivery of quality care.

The benefits
There are two main benefits of clinical supervision:

- **Improved patient care and satisfaction**
  This can be achieved in a number of ways:

  - monitoring of practice – the opportunity for practice to be monitored by regular discussion between the nurse and the supervisor to underpin accountability.
  - reflection on practice – the opportunity to examine and evaluate episodes and incidents from practice.
  - development of practice – the identification of developmental needs for individual nurses and the organisation.

- **Development of potential**
  This will include development of:

  - the individual – to use and extend their clinical skills;
  - the organisation – to have effective staff with the opportunity to develop their practice;
  - the profession – by having a nursing workforce that is regularly examining and developing its practice.

Supervision may also contribute to a number of additional issues related to clinical practice:

- It may help to reduce sick leave among nurses.
- It can help appraisal by identifying clinically based goals and by providing regular evaluation of existing goals.

cont'd

BOX 6.6 (cont'd)

- It can help nurses to identify their educational and training needs.
- It can help to develop constructive dialogue between staff, improve communications and help to develop teamwork.
- It can increase work satisfaction and improve retention and recruitment.
- It can help nurses to cope with professional demands and expectations.

The principal functions
There are three principal functions of clinical supervision that are mutually inclusive. It is essential that all three are considered during clinical supervision. This will prevent it becoming managerial control, a tutorial or a counselling session. The three functions are:

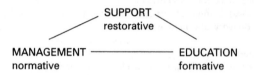

These are the terms used by Kadushin (1976) and Proctor (1991), and will help the nurse by:

- giving support to cope with the demands of developing and exploring practice;
- offering a managerial perspective to situations and experiences that the nurse encounters;
- providing new information and identifying educational opportunities.

Modes of supervision
The following aspects of the supervision process should be clearly considered in advance of commencing clinical supervision:

- *Where* – it is essential that privacy and time are provided for supervision. It should be a rostered activity that is identified as an essential aspect of the nurses' work.
- *When* – it is suggested that this should be agreed by the nurses involved but should be at least every 8 weeks, for approximately 40 minutes.
- *Who* – to avoid bottlenecks and overload, no one nurse should be responsible for providing supervision for more than 6 colleagues. Every nurse should be provided individual supervision and, if possible, group/peer supervision. Nurses offering supervision to others should be in supervision themselves.

cont'd

BOX 6.6 (cont'd)

The following three dimensions offer a number of options for deciding who should provide the supervision:

1 *Which profession?*
   – own;
   – other, e.g. psychology, medicine;
   – more than one.

2 *What level, or grade of staff?*
   – higher;
   – peer;
   – both.

3 *What number of staff?*
   – one-to-one;
   – group;
   – both.

If it is not a more senior nurse who provides the individual supervision, it is suggested that the choice of supervisor should meet the approval of the nurse's line manager.

- *Records*
  The records of clinical supervision should be kept confidentially by individual nurses in their personal professional profiles. The use of learning contracts to record supervisory activity is one method of ensuring that needs are formalised. Records of the supervision events may be held by the supervisor to monitor the practice.

Dangers to clinical supervision
There are a number of potential dangers to the process of clinical supervision:

- self-congratulation and short-sightedness;
- domination of the process by the supervisor;
- domination of the process by organisational needs;
- linkage of supervision to performance-related pay;
- operation of supervision in isolation from appraisal;
- a prescriptive approach to the process;
- consensus collusion;
- operation as confessional or counselling.

Skills of the supervisor
A number of skills of the supervisor will assist in ensuring that the process is developmental:

cont'd

BOX 6.6 (cont'd)

- listening in a safe environment to the nurse's practice development agenda;
- questioning to explore and clarify the nurse's practice and understanding;
- analysis and the provision of feedback to explore practice (reflection);
- facilitation and confrontation to help development proceed;
- sensitivity to the needs of the organisation.

Requirements of the supervisee
A number of features from the supervisee will facilitate the process:

- the identification of practice issues;
- preparedness to share these experiences;
- considering feedback and discriminating upon its value;
- the readiness to change practice in the light of exploration.

Summary
There is no one right way to operate clinical supervision, but it essential that agreement is reached on the following aspects:

- the introduction of clinical supervision by local facilitation and not as a management proposition or decree;
- the purpose of clinical supervision;
- the process of that clinical supervision;
- the relationship between supervision and appraisal;
- the relationship between supervision and management functions, such as performance-related pay and disciplinary action;
- clarification between clinical supervision and the statutory supervision of midwives;
- the means by which clinical supervision will be evaluated and reviewed to ensure it is meeting the needs of the nurses;
- the degree of confidentiality – absolute or negotiated.

Bibliography
Bishop, V. 1994 Clinical supervision for an accountable profession. *Nursing Times* **90**(39): 35–7.
Hawkins, P and Shohet, R. 1989 *Supervision in the Helping Professions*. Milton Keynes: Open University Press.
Kadushin, A. 1976 *Supervision in Social Work*. New York: Columbia University Press.
Kohner, N. 1994 *Clinical Supervision: an Executive Summary*. London: King's Fund Centre.
Procter, B. (1991) Supervision: a co-operative exercise in accountability. In Marken, M. and Payne, M. (eds) *Enabling and Ensuring*. Leicestershire: National Youth Bureau and Council for Education and Training in Youth and Community Work.

cont'd

BOX 6.6 (cont'd)

Acknowledgement
These guidelines were generated from work as the clinical leader of the King's Fund-supported Nursing Development Unit (NDU), John Radcliffe Hospital Oxford, and from research that looked at 'Appraisal and Professional Fulfilment for Nurses'. The latter case study revealed that many nurses were uncertain about the answer, and dissatisfied with their experiences of appraisal. These guidelines reflect their views about clinical supervision as an activity to support appraisal as a means to develop nurses. They also reflect the experiences of introducing clinical supervision onto the NDU and elsewhere.

References

Adair, L. and Murray, L. 1995 Organisation of Nursing Care project: Nursing Development Unit (King's Fund) John Radcliffe Hospital Oxford. In Bowman, G. and Thompson, D. (eds) *A Classification System for Nurses' Work Methods: The Bowman Classification*. Oxford: National Institute of Nursing.

Bennis, W. and Nanus, B. 1985 *Leaders*. New York: Harper & Row.

Block, P. 1993 *Stewardship*. San Francisco: Berrett-Koehler.

Brookfield, S. 1987 *Developing Critical Thinkers*. Milton Keynes: Open University Press.

Butterworth, T. and Faugier J. 1992 *Clinical Supervision*. London: Chapman & Hall.

Cooper, C. 1988 Stress, mental health and job satisfaction. *Health Service Management Research* **1**(1).

Corder, L. 1996 Level the playing field. *Nursing Times* **96**(9): 30–2.

Daloz, L. 1987 *Effective Teaching and Mentoring*. San Francisco: Jossey-Bass.

Ersser, S. and Tutton E. 1991 *Primary Nursing in Perspective*. London: Scutari Press.

Garbett, R. 1992 Attested development. *Nursing Times* **88**(35): 40–1.

Garbett, R. 1993 Your choice. *Nursing Times* **89**(17): 49–51.

Garbett, R. 1994 Changing philosophy through group interview: a flexible tool in nursing development. *Nursing Development News* **7**: 3–4.

Handy, C. 1994 *The Empty Raincoat*. London: Arrow Books.

Hawkins, P. and Shohet, R. 1989 *Supervision in the Helping Professions*. Milton Keynes: Open University Press.

Hingley, P. and Harris, P. 1986 Burnout at senior level. *Nursing Times* **82**(32): 52–3.

Kohner, N. 1994a *Clinical Supervision in Practice*. London: King's Fund Centre/Poole: BEBC.

Kohner, N. 1994b *Clinical Supervision: an Executive Summary.* London: King's Fund Centre.

Marcellison, F., Winnubusts, J., Buunk, B. and De Wolff, C. 1988 Social support and occupational stress. *Social Science and Medicine* **26**(3): 365–73.

Maslach, C. 1982 *Burnout: The Cost of Caring.* New Jersey: Prentice-Hall.

Mezirow, J. 1981 A critical theory of adult learning and education. *Adult Education* **32**(1): 3–24.

National Health Service Training Authority 1986 *Guide and Model Documentation for Individualised Performance Review.* Bristol: NHSTA.

Northcott, N. 1994 Organisational culture in a nursing development unit. *Nursing Review* **12**(3 & 4): 12–14.

Northcott, N. 1996a *Appraisal and Professional Fulfilment of Nursing Staff in Oxfordshire.* Unpublished thesis. Southampton: University of Southampton.

Northcott, N. 1996b The significance of culture in an NDU. *Nursing Developments News* **15**: 3–5.

Northcott, N. 1996c Contracts for good morale. *Nursing Management* **3**(3): 23.

Pedlar, M., Burgoyne, J. and Boydell, T. 1991 *The Learning Company.* New York: McGraw Hill.

Scholes, J. 1996 Staff role transition and emotional labour in nursing development units. *Nursing Times* **92**(31): 40–42.

UKCC (United Kingdom Central Council for Nursing, Midwifery and Health Visiting) 1990 *The Post-Registration Education and Practice Project.* London: UKCC.

UKCC (United Kingdom Central Council for Nursing, Midwifery and Health Visiting) 1992a *Scope of Professional Practice.* London: UKCC.

UKCC (United Kingdom Central Council for Nursing, Midwifery and Health Visiting) 1992b *Code of Professional Conduct.* London: UKCC.

UKCC (United Kingdom Central Council for Nursing, Midwifery and Health Visiting) 1996 *Position Paper on Clinical Supervision for Nursing and Health Visiting.* London: UKCC.

Usher, R. and Edwards, R. 1994 *Postmodernism and Education.* London: Routledge.

Vaughan, B. 1989 Developing trends in nursing. In Vaughan, B. and Pilmoor, M. (eds) *Managing Nursing Work.* London: Scutari Press.

Whitehead, L. 1989 Taking the strain. In Vaughan, B. and Pilmoor, M. (eds) *Managing Nursing Work.* London: Scutari Press.

Wolfgang, A. 1988 Job stress in health professions. *Behavioural Medicine* **14**(1): 43–7.

7

Towards Effective Training of Clinical Supervisors

Chris Scanlon

Despite a broad consensus that clinical supervision is essentially a psycho-educational activity, very little has been written to date by nurse teachers about how best to prepare practitioners for its more widespread implementation. This chapter describes some of the contextual issues relating to practitioner knowledge and nurse education, and their application to effective clinical supervision practices. Focus is on the educational requirements of both supervisees and of supervisors, and some specific suggestions are offered on how such training could be managed.

Practitioner knowledge and nurse education

What do we mean by 'knowledge'? In attempting to provide a philosophical underpinning for nurse education, both Benner and Wrubel (1982) and Burnard (1987) have made the distinction between two domains of knowledge, previously described as 'knowing that' and 'knowing how'. Heron (1996) describes practice-based knowledge as 'having the knack'. Viewed from this perspective, practice is not merely the application of theory but is grounded in a third, deeply subjective, domain of 'personal knowledge' (Polanyi, 1967). In the specific context of nursing, this personal knowledge is described by Meerabeau (1992) as tacit nursing knowledge. The regrettably poor relationship between 'theoretical education' and 'training for practice' has been explored by Jarvis (1992), and research within nursing has shown the extent to which an overevaluation of the technical–rational approach in nurse education adversely effects practice, recent examples being McCaugherty (1991) and Conway (1994). Against this background, Johns (1995) suggests that the reflective practice model outlined by Schon (1987) might offer an ideal method to structure clinical supervision in order to ensure that practice and theory become better integrated.

Truly skilled practitioners are those who involve themselves in a 'reflective conversation with the situation' (Schon, 1983, p. 68) in which they are not dependent on established theory and technique, which separates thinking from doing, but rather construct a 'theory of the unique case' with which they are more personally engaged. This process that Schon termed 'reflection-in-action' has been extensively drawn upon and has formed the basis for an important and growing critical evaluation of practices within nursing (Atkins and Murphy, 1993; Conway, 1994; Johns, 1995). In Schon's view, although such developments can be 'coached', they cannot be taught in the formal sense and instead require a different context and different facilitation skills from those normally associated with teaching in higher education. In nursing, these 'coaching' skills have also been referred to as 'mentoring' skills (Butterworth, 1992), the skills of the 'teacher-practitioner' (Knight, 1992), preceptorship skills (Ashton and Richardson, 1992) and, more recently, the skills of the clinical supervisor (Hawkins and Shohet, 1989; Butterworth and Faugier, 1992).

The supervisory relationship

Hawkins and Shohet (1989) suggest that the practitioner–supervisor relationship has several different foci that indirectly parallel Schon's distinction between 'reflection-*on*-action' and the higher order skill of 'reflection-*in*-action' described above. The former type of reflection, which allows practitioners to learn interpersonal skills by thinking about past actions, has been extensively researched under the very broad description of 'experiential learning' (Heron, 1992) and has been widely used in interpersonal skills training in nurse education (Burnard, 1995). While there is little doubt that such 'reflection-on-action' is often helpful in more conscious problem-solving, it may be suggested that such a retrospective analysis is also limited because it is dependent on what practitioners *can* articulate about their practice rather than what they *cannot* (Greenwood, 1993).

Some practical issues

The UKCC (1996) has clearly stated that it wants to see a component of pre- and post-registration education and training dedicated to preparing practitioners to *receive* clinical supervision. However, very little guidance has been issued with regard to the prerequisite level or kind of training necessary to *provide* effective clinical supervision. Instead, this decision of setting criteria for defining who will be a supervisor has been left to local service providers. Butterworth *et al.* (1996) suggest this has resulted in a tension between a desire for a top-down imposition of directives for the role of *clinical* supervisors from the UKCC and the wish to train clinical supervisors in a way that is more responsive to local need. The result is that there is now widespread confusion and disagreement. This often revolves around pragmatic difficulties, such as the cost of training clinical supervisors, rather than around issues of what constitutes best practice. Unfortunately, nursing literature offers little guidance here. In the hope of remedying this situation, I shall now recount my own experience of attempting to provide preparatory training for supervisees and more specific training aiming to prepare practitioners to undertake the role of clinical supervisor. In the next section, I shall describe what I consider to be some of the crucial issues in effective training for practice and offer some tentative suggestions for a possible way forward.

Educating supervisees

As with any attempt to influence a cultural change, and the use of clinical supervision in nursing with its drive for personal and collective empowerment and change, it is first necessary to raise people's consciousness about the extent to which they are disempowered. Rafferty and Coleman (1995) suggest that this might be facilitated by offering a rolling programme of 'in-house', half-day workshops that all staff could attend. To be effective, such training clearly requires some investment of time and money, and the employment of a skilled facilitator to undertake the training. However, it is anticipated that, as training for clinical supervision becomes better integrated into existing preregistration and specialist post-registration clinical courses, the need for this type of 'in-house' preparatory training will lessen and eventually be phased out.

Many Trusts have already begun the journey by holding initial informal meetings with the 'movers and shakers' within their clinical staff, and have then cascaded this discussion into a wider forum such as through a conference with invited external speakers with expertise on the subject. It is essential, if change is to be effected – particularly in large organisations with competing pressures – to ensure some degree of ownership of the new direction, and obtaining some consensus statement may be seen as crucial to achieve this. This can be obtained in various ways, but an interactive process is necessary, as is a timetable to which key people are signed up that will help to identify the shared goals and promote their delivery. One of the most difficult tasks is to maintain the initial enthusiasm engendered by the successful introduction of the concept of clinical supervision, and careful planning will be needed to ensure that a rosy promise does not become dirtied by apathy.

In such short workshops it is clearly necessary to avoid over-complicated theory in favour of a critical discussion of the structure of the supervisory process. My own practice is to use a structural diagram (Figure 7.1) adapted from the double-matrix model of Hawkins and Shohet (1989). Using this model, the practitioner is 'placed' in the centre of the matrix and clinical supervision is proposed as a 'nurse-centred model for nursing'. Thus the general foci for discussion, corresponding to the numbers on the diagram, are

1   the *affective* nature of being a patient in terms of vulnerability, need, pain, suffering, loss, death, stigma and joy;

2   the *affecting* nature of being compassionately in relation to
    patients, and the adaptive and maladaptive coping
    mechanisms used to defend against anxiety arising out of
    these relationships;
3   the *acute* and *cumulative* cost of being a caring nurse in terms
    of occupational stress and burnout (Maslach, 1981; Booth,
    1992);
4   the supervisory relationship; *supportive, formative* and
    normative functions (Proctor, 1986) and some discussion of
    the dynamic of the *parallel process* (Hawkins and Shohet,
    1989; Bramley, 1996);
5   the qualities of the supervisory relationship and the
    implications for training;
6   clinical supervision contrasted with quality issues linked to
    patients–clinical audit, and so on;
7   clinical supervision contrasted with staff appraisal systems;
    horizontal versus vertical authority in staff development
    (Platt-Koch, 1986; Butterworth, 1992; UKCC, 1996);
8   the relationship of the clinical supervisor to the management
    systems, for example the parameters of confidentiality,
    resourcing issues, contracting, prerequisite criteria, and so on.

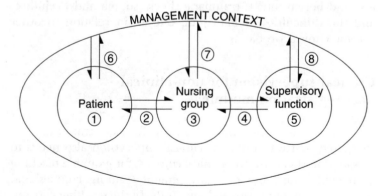

Figure 7.1   The supervising matrix

Clinical supervision for specialist post-registration clinical courses

The UKCC (1996) clearly states that an introduction to 'the principles and relevance of clinical supervision' should be an integrated and compulsory core component on all post-registration clinical courses. The amount of time given over to clinical supervision should not be prescribed and standardised for all courses; however, it is suggested that such decisions are reached collaboratively with a teacher or practitioner skilled in clinical supervision rather than left to specialist module leaders to decide. This offers an important precedent in the establishment of a collaborative relationship between specialist practitioner and clinical supervisor in a way which reflects the cultural shift that the students themselves are being asked to make.

In the next few years, with the concept of clinical supervision still in its infancy, it is suggested that input on clinical supervision might begin with a general discussion of the issues such as described in the 'in-house' training outlined above. This discussion could then be extended to examine in more depth the particular clinical problems presented by working in a particular clinical environment and how they may become a focus within clinical supervision, for example, managing the particular frustrations of chronic illness, infirmity and decline, loss and bereavement, traumatic shock, stigma and prejudice, and the difficulties of managing oneself in relation to other specific clinical problems.

Clinical supervision for non-clinical post-registration modules

In addition to input into clinically focused training, it is suggested that the profile of clinical supervision also needs to be raised in specialist non-clinical courses, for example teaching and mentorship courses, management training courses and courses in qualitative research methods. In the teaching courses, the content could be adapted to compare and contrast clinical supervision with other experiential learning processes such as self- and peer-assessment strategies, role modelling, mentor-

ship and preceptorship. In the management training programmes, content would compare and contrast clinical supervision with specific staff appraisal systems and discuss the place
of clinical supervision in the maintenance of professional and
ethical issues (Johns, 1993a, b; Bramley, 1996; Barker and
Davidson, 1997) and the management of change (Hooker, 1991;
Obholzer and Roberts, 1994; Hart, 1996).

The qualitative research methods course could present for
critique clinical supervision as a reflexive research tool for
getting at 'tacit knowledge embedded in practice' (Meerbeau,
1992). This critique may be extended to include a discussion
of the place of reflexive approaches in general, for example
in the use of an action research methodology (Greenwood,
1994; Hart, 1996) or an approach calling upon so-called natu-
ralistic and new paradigm research methods (Meyer, 1993).
This might also include a discussion about the similarities and
differences between the process of clinical and research supervision when attempting to make use of these more qualitative approaches.

Changing the culture through nurse teachers

As has been clearly illustrated by Melia (1987), the forces of
occupational socialisation in nursing are both influential and
pervasive, and begin from the start of training. Indeed, such
is the importance of this issue that the UKCC (1996) states
that the principles and relevance of clinical supervision should
begin in preregistration education. Schon (1987) argues that
one of the difficulties of establishing *any* training for practitioner education within university departments is the difference in status between those who 'teach and/or develop' theory
and those who facilitate learning from practice. One of the major
problems, he suggests, is that staff members, even if they are
to be employed to facilitate interpersonal skills developments,
are appointed on the basis of their academic qualifications
alone rather than in recognition of their training in experiential learning methods or clinical supervision. Given these
concerns, Schon (1987, p. 171) stresses that the 'reflective practice' approach to professional education would not survive as

a second-class activity. He goes on to suggest that one of the most important ways of influencing the culture of professional education is for facilitators of knowledgeable learning from practice to be seen to be first-class members of university departments. This priority must be reflected in the recruitment and selection of staff to undertake these roles.

One possible solution to this problem is more widespread appointment of lecturer–practitioners (Knight, 1992) and/or practitioner–researchers (Greenwood, 1994) who would be jointly funded by health service and educational providers. Such joint appointments are only practical if the 'education and training' and/or 'research and development' aspect and the practitioner role are very specifically defined so that the post-holder is able to spend sufficient time in direct patient contact in order to be, and be seen to be, a credible practitioner.

It must be understood that clinical supervision requires clearly planned intervention by skilled practitioners with advanced training in individual, group and organisation dynamics and that to train such people requires an investment of time and money. Against this background, I agree with Faugier and Butterworth (1995) that it is probably unrealistic, in the short term at least, not to seek to make creative use of interprofessional supervision by and/or with other multidisciplinary team members who have more experience of offering training in clinical supervision. Indeed, Skynner (1989) describes a positive advantage of this interprofessional co-operation in terms of what he called the 'emperor's new clothes phenomenon,' whereby the outsider can often ask the apparently naive questions that a practitioner embedded in that culture may not yet be able to see. In a recent review of NHS psychotherapy services, the NHSE recommended that psychotherapists should have a role in providing consultancy and support to help all staff develop a reflective approach to practice (Parry and Richardson, 1996). It might well be that there is also a great deal of scope for suitably qualified counsellors and psychotherapists *within* nursing to take a lead in offering education and training for clinical supervision.

Training specifications

In order to underline the importance of clinical supervision and to enable appropriate levels of supervisory skill, I suggest that training should be part time and extend over a sufficient period to allow for the necessary skills to develop. However, given the urgent need to establish 'good enough' rather than ideal training, it may be necessary, in the interim, to combine the training for supervisees and for clinical supervisors by some degree of shared learning. This could be achieved by dividing the training into two parts.

The first part would be open to all practitioners and would as such *not* be seen as a training for supervisors but rather as an introduction to the art and science of clinical supervision. Rafferty and Coleman (1995) describe a well-evaluated day-release module extending over a 3-month period, approved by the Welsh National Board and offered at undergraduate diploma level (level 2), which might serve as a model for such an introduction. However, I would contend that a sufficiently in-depth understanding of the theoretical and practical issues involved in the supervisory process requires a capacity for critical analysis that could not reasonably be expected of a practitioner undertaking level 2 studies.

The second part of the training, although building on the first, would be a selective training for clinical supervisors only and would probably need to be offered at a higher academic level.

Selection of practitioners for training as clinical supervisors

Sharpe (1995a) suggests, in the related field of group psychotherapy, that any supervisor training that seeks to train all-comers is probably defensively avoiding the uncomfortable problem of deciding which practitioners are best cut out to do it. In this context, the following criteria are suggested as the minimum prerequisites for specialist training in clinical supervision:

- a minimum of 2 years' clinical experience with at least some degree of specialisation within a particular area of practice;
- good evidence of motivation towards raising and maintaining professional standards, including working in a clearly defined mentorship role with health care assistants and/or students;
- clear evidence of ongoing professional development, as demonstrated by the presentation of a coherent and recent education and training portfolio;
- good interpersonal skills;
- a capacity to be with people under stress, demonstrated by a clear exposition of personal strategies for understanding and responding to one's own sources of stress and anxiety;
- a capacity to work effectively in a team, demonstrated through having managed staff and/or users of services in a clearly defined clinical setting.

It could be argued that many nurses demonstrate their capacity to meet these criteria daily. In addition, it is suggested that the prospective trainee would need to be in a post within which he or she would be actually able to offer clinical supervision, preferably under the supervision of a more experienced clinical supervisor. In this role, trainee supervisors would need to have sufficient knowledge and experience of practice to be able to be confident in their professional authority. Realistically, this would mean a practitioner who is at a minimum level of a clinical grade F and optimally at grade G or equivalent.

Training of supervisors

Almost all commentators agree that, to be an effective clinical supervisor, it is necessary first to be both an expert practitioner and then to have had a 'good enough' experience of clinical supervision oneself (Hawkins and Shohet, 1989; Sharpe, 1995; Carroll, 1996). Similarly, most agree that, even when available, such an experience is not in itself sufficient fully to appreciate the complexities of the supervisory relationship and that there needs to be clearly designated specialist training for supervisors. However, one of the most pressing issues facing professional leaders and health service managers alike is to decide what the professional status of the clinical supervisor in nursing is to be. Following on from this, the difficult question for the teacher is to know at what academic and/or professional level to present training for such a role. In discussing this issue, Wright (1992) compared the supervisory role for nursing with the role and function of a consultant in medicine and suggested, therefore, that such a consultant nurse would not only need to have advanced standing as a practitioner, but would also need to be educated at least to Masters degree level. This new role would then become part of the vanguard of what of Salvage (1990) describes as the politics of 'new nursing" and might also reward senior and experienced staff to remain in clinical practice rather than to seek career development in an academic or managerial capacity (Wright, 1992).

There has to date been very little specific work outlining the learning needs of clinical supervisors in nursing. However, within a wider professional literature (Hawkins and Shohet, 1989; Carroll, 1996), there is a general consensus that training clinical supervisors would have a number of key ingredients that I have modified and adapted for the specific cultural context of nursing. It may well be that each branch of nursing would have differing ideas about which of these components would form the core of any such training opportunity. Any approach to the training of clinical supervisors must be firmly underpinned by an informed critique of the interpersonal, psychodynamic and psychosocial models outlined above. For the convenience of the reader and ease of presentation, the proposed content is divided into the theoretical issues that would be included in a more general introductory module and more specialist theoretical issues, appended at the end of this chapter, that would need to be addressed in the more advanced training. Selected reference material is included as a further guide to the territory.

Training for practice

To be able to bring about the necessary cultural change in nursing for effective clinical supervision, I suggest that the supervisor should have 'good enough' initial understanding of the group and organisational dynamic that might enhance or limit such a development. This is not to suggest that group supervision is always the choice for conducting clinical supervision, and indeed, whichever model is selected, be it one-to-one or group supervision, it must suit the individuals and the resources of the locality concerned. Rather it is a statement about the need for the supervisor to feel comfortable in a group and thus make links between the individual practitioner and his or her social and organisational context. Clearly, one of the best ways to learn about group process is to have the experience of being in a group.

One group model that has proved very versatile in enabling practitioners to learn from practice is the so-called Balint 'work discussion groups' (Balint *et al.*, 1993), pioneered at the Tavistock clinic. These groups are designed to offer experiential support and raise awareness of psychosocial and interpersonal issues arising from the practitioners' work; they have been used to good effect in the training of a wide range of health and social care professionals. As shown by Franks *et al.* (1994), experiential groups, properly conducted, also enable practitioners to feel supported and develop increased self-confidence, and enhance interpersonal skill development. As Bray (1997) suggests, this increased confidence and greater capacity to reflect on the challenges of work may even then lead into a more sophisticated collective reflection-in-action on deeper personal and political problems, which may then lead to shifts in the cultural matrix of nursing-as-a-whole.

Given that nursing is essentially a team/group-based activity, I would argue that the only way in which nursing-as-a-whole can be allowed to change in the long term is through the informed and skilful use of reflective groups. To develop the skills and confidence to conduct reflective groups of this type is, however, a long and difficult process and requires specific training above and beyond that which is possible to develop in the training programmes outlined above. It is perhaps worth noting, however, that, apart from isolated pockets of activity, for example within the therapeutic communities movement, there is very little specific training in group work offered by nurses for nurses. Thus, if nursing wishes to evolve into a more reflective culture, I would argue that we must also consider how we might train practitioners to be able to consult confidently with whole staff teams. Indeed, I would suggest that the lack of specific group facilitator training is a serious problem that can only hinder the development of a true culture of inquiry within nursing.

For an effective training, it will also be clearly understood that trainee clinical supervisors must have logged a specified minimum number of hours in developing their skills in practice. The extent to which the trainee is best developed by being encouraged to offer x number of hours to several different practitioners and thus to encounter a wide range of different practitioners' problems versus a strategy in which the practitioner is encouraged to pay close attention to the process of working with a smaller number of subjects remains an interesting one, which Scanlon and Baillie (1994) suggest deserves to be further researched.

Assessment strategies

In proposing a more reflective approach to practice, Schon (1987) calls not only for new, 'practice-led' curricula, but also for a new way of assessing learning that is more in keeping with this approach. He does not, however, suggest that the assessment of theoretical understanding is abandoned altogether, but rather argues for a redefinition of the relationship between theory and practice so that, rather than merely focus on the science of nursing, we should make better use of the art involved in the provision of good care. To achieve this, it is suggested that assessment might have two interrelated components: first, some assessment of this art of skilful 'doing', and second, an assessment of the theory underpinning this skilful doing. Theoretical assessment would need to demonstrate the capacity to link aspects of their practice to underpinning and/or overarching theory. They would, however, need to be practice-led rather than theory-driven. This would require there to be an in-depth analysis of the content and process of the supervisory relationship in the context of a clearly defined model for supervision. One approach that proved to be very successful in the training of a wide range of health professionals is that of interpersonal process recall (O'Callaghan and Cowie, 1995). Using this technique, the process and content of a series of supervision sessions could be audio- and/or videotape recorded and evaluated by the trainee and his or her peer group using a modified self- and peer-assessment strategy (Kilty, 1978). The trainee supervisors would ideally themselves be supervised on this work by a more experienced supervisor, who would then be in a position to assess the trainees' development.

With a greater availability of experienced supervisors, there may also increasingly be the possibility for conjoint live supervision, which would involve the trainee supervisor co-working *in situ* with a more experienced supervisor in a group supervision session, a method frequently used to good effect in the training of family and group therapists. However, given the shortage of sufficiently experienced supervisors, it might well be that, in the interim, this role would fall to the module teacher.

Conclusion

In this chapter, I have outlined contextual issues surrounding clinical supervision and its application to nursing practice across all disciplines. While sympathetic to the need for a degree of pragmatism in the initial implementation of clinical supervision and the use of in-house expertise, I have emphasised the need for grounded theory and for advanced education and training in the development of the role of the supervisor within the context of higher education. An important factor to consider is the cultural change required for realising the benefits of effective clinical supervision. To achieve this, it is essential to involve some degree of learning with all staff involved.

I would like to thank Dr Geraldine Byrne (University of Hertfordshire), Mr Ben Davidson (Pathfinder NHS Trust), Dr Julienne Meyer (City University), Ms Lynny Turner (City University), Mrs Amanda Weir (Henderson Hospital), Mr Joe Weir (University of Surrey), Mrs Dianne Yarwood (City University) and my friends and colleagues at the Institute of Group Analysis (London) for their encouragement during the writing of this chapter. The work is dedicated to the memory of my former colleague Claire Virgo.

Appendix

Introduction to the art and science of clinical supervision

- Defining clinical supervision and contrasting it with other enabling processes such as mentorship, preceptorship and management appraisal systems (Platt-Koch, 1986; Butterworth, 1992).
- Theoretical knowledge about different models of supervision (Hawkins and Shohet, 1989).
- Understanding of the different roles and functions of the supervisor, teacher, consultant, researcher, mentor and evaluator (Peplau, 1952; Travelbee, 1971).
- The reflective practitioner in nursing (Powell, 1989; Saylor, 1990; Greenwood, 1993; Johns, 1995).
- The nature of clinical knowledge (Benner and Wrubel, 1982; Burnard, 1987; Meerabeau, 1992).
- The stages and phases of the process of clinical supervision and the supervisory relationship (Faugier, 1992; Carroll, 1996).
- Occupational stress and burnout (Maslach, 1981; Booth, 1992).
- Social functioning as a defence against anxiety (Menzies, 1959; Obholzer and Roberts, 1994).
- Introduction to the group process (Wright, 1989; Franks *et al.*, 1994).

Further training for clinical supervisors

- The therapeutic relationship revisited to include a critical analysis of the complex *unconscious* processes that distort interpersonal effectiveness (Fabricius, 1991, 1995; Wright, 1991; Dartington, 1994; Bray, 1997).
- The psychosocial construction of the 'unpopular patient' (Stockwell, 1972; Kelly and May, 1982; Johnson and Webb, 1995).
- Holding and containing in the parallel process (Wright, 1991; Dartington, 1994; James, 1994; Bramley, 1996).
- Working with interpersonal resistance to clinical supervision (Bramley, 1996; Bray, 1997).

- Ethical decision-making in practice (Johns, 1993a, b; Bramley, 1996; Barker and Davidson, 1997).
- An understanding of cultural differences influencing supervisory process such as power, gender, sociocultural difference and ethnicity (Carpio and Majumdar, 1993; Carroll, 1996).
- Constructive and destructive forces in groups (Ernst and Goodison, 1981; Wright 1989; Franks *et al.*, 1994).
- Organisational action research, staff team consultation and the management of change (Bowman, 1986; Hooker, 1991; Obholzer and Roberts 1994; Hart, 1996).
- The concept of a self-generating, peer-learning community (Heron, 1974, 1978), learning organisation (Argyris and Schon, 1978) or culture of inquiry (Chapman, 1984; Barber, 1988).

References

Argyris, C. and Schon, D. A. 1978 *Organisational Learning*. London: Addison-Wesley.

Ashton, P. and Richardson, G. 1992 Preceptorship and PREP. *British Journal of Nursing* **1**(3): 143–5.

Atkins, S. and Murphy, K. 1993 Reflection: a review of the literature. *Journal of Advanced Nursing* **18**(8): 1188–92.

Balint, E., Courtenay, M., Elder, A., Hull, S. and Julian, P. 1993 *The Doctor, the Patient and the Group*. London: Routledge.

Barber, P. 1988 Learning to grow: the necessity for educational processing in the therapeutic community practice. *International Journal of Therapeutic Communities* **9**: 101–8.

Barker, P. and Davidson, B. 1997 *Psychiatric Nursing: Ethical Strife*. London: Edward Arnold.

Benner, P. and Wrubel, J. 1982 Skilled clinical knowledge; the values of perceptual awareness. *Nurse Educator* May/June: 11–17.

Booth, K. 1992 Providing support and reducing stress: a review of the literature. In: Butterworth, T. and Faugier, J. (eds) *Clinical Supervision and Mentorship in Nursing*. London: Chapman Hall.

Bowman, M. P. 1986 *Nursing Management and Education: A Conceptual Approach to Change*. London: Croom-Helm.

Bramley, W. 1996 *The Supervisory Couple in Broad Spectrum Psychotherapy*. London: Free Association Press.

Bray, J. 1997 Psychiatric nursing and the myth of altruism. In: Barker, P. and Davidson, B. (eds) *Psychiatric Nursing: Ethical Strife*, London: Edward Arnold.

Burnard, P. 1987 Towards an epistemological basis for nurse education. *Journal of Advanced Nursing* **12**: 189–93.

Burnard, P. 1995 *Learning Human Skills. An Experiential and Reflective Guide for Nurses*, 3rd edn. London: Heinemann.

Butterworth, T. 1992 Clinical supervision as an emerging idea in nursing. In: Butterworth, T. and Faugier, J. (eds) *Clinical Supervision and Mentorship in Nursing*. London: Chapman & Hall.

Butterworth, T. and Faugier, J. (1992) *Clinical Supervision and Mentorship in Nursing*. London: Chapman & Hall.

Butterworth, T., Bishop, V. and Carson, J. 1996 First steps towards evaluating clinical supervision in nursing and health visiting: theory, policy and practice developments. *Journal of Clinical Nursing* **5**: 127–32.

Carpio, B.A. and Mujumdar, B. 1993 Experiential learning: an approach to transcultural education for nursing. *Journal of Transcultural Nursing* **4**: 4–11.

Carroll, M. 1996 *Counselling Supervision. Theory, Skills and Practice*. London: Cassell.

Chapman, G.E. 1984 A therapeutic community, psychosocial nursing and the nursing process. *International Journal of Therapeutic Communities* **5**: 68–76.

Conway, J. 1994 Reflection, the art and science of nursing and the theory–practice gap. *British Journal of Nursing* **3**(3): 114–18.

Dartington, A. 1994 Where angels fear to tread – idealism, despondency, and inhibition in thought in hospital nursing. In: Obholzer, A. and Roberts, V.Z. (eds) *The Unconscious at Work. Individual and Organisational Stress in the Human Services*. London: Routledge.

Ernst, S. and Goodison, L. 1981 *In Our Own Hands: A Book of Self Help Therapy*. London: Heinemann.

Fabricius, J. 1991 Running on the spot or can nursing really change. *Psychoanalytic Psychotherapy* **5**(2): 97–108.

Fabricius, J. 1995 Psychoanalytic understanding and nursing – a supervisory workshop with nurse tutors. *Psychoanalytic Psychotherapy* **9**: 17–29.

Faugier, J. 1992 The supervisory relationship in clinical supervision. In: Butterworth, T. and Faugier, J. (eds) *Clinical Supervision and Mentorship in Nursing*. London: Chapman & Hall.

Faugier, J. and Butterworth, T. 1995 Clinical supervision: a position paper. In: *Clinical Supervision – a Resource Pack*. London: NHS Management Executive.

Franks, V., Watts, M. and Fabricius, J. 1994 Interpersonal learning in groups: an investigation. *Journal of Advanced Nursing* **20**: 1162–9.

Greenwood, J. 1993 Reflective practice: a critique of the work of Argyris and Schon. *Journal of Advanced Nursing* **18**(8): 1183–7.

Greenwood J. 1994 Action research: a few details, a caution and something new. *Journal of Advanced Nursing* **20**(1): 13–18.

Hart, E. 1996 Action research as a professionalising strategy. *Journal of Advanced Nursing* **23**: 454–61.

Hawkins, P. and Shohet, R. 1989 *Supervision in the Helping Professions*. Milton Keynes: Open University Press.

Heron, J. 1974 *The Peer Learning Community*. Guildford: University of Surrey Press.

Heron, J. 1978 *Project for a Self-generating Culture*. Guildford: University of Surrey.

Heron, J. 1992 *Feeling and Personhood. Psychology in Another Key*. London: Sage.

Heron, J. 1996 Quality as primacy of practical. *Qualitative Inquiry* **2**(1): 41–57.

Hooker, J.C. 1991 Change and nursing in the United Kingdom. *Journal of Advanced Nursing* **16**: 253–4.

James, D.C. 1994 Holding and containing in the group and in society. In: Brown, D. and Zinkin, L.M. (eds) *The Psyche and the Social World. Developments in Group-Analytic Theory*. London: Routledge.

Jarvis, P. 1993 Quality in practice; the role of education. *Nurse Education Today* 12: 2–10.

Johns, C. 1993a On becoming effective in taking ethical actions. *Journal of Clinical Nursing* **2**: 307–12.

Johns, C. 1993b Professional supervision. *Journal of Nursing Management* **1**: 9–18.

Johns, C. 1995 The value of reflective practice for nursing. *Journal of Clinical Nursing* **4**: 23–30.

Johnson, M. and Webb, C. 1995 Rediscovering unpopular patients: the concept of social judgement. *Journal of Advanced Nursing* **21**(3): 466–75.

Kilty, J. 1978 *Self and Peer Assessment*. Human Potential Research Project. Guildford: University of Surrey.

Kelly, M.P. and May, D. 1982 Good and bad patients: a review of the literature and a theoretical critique. *Journal of Advanced Nursing* **7**: 147–56.

Knight, J. 1992 The lecturer-practitioner role: an exploration and reflection. *Journal of Clinical Nursing* **1**: 58–9.

McCaugherty, D. 1991 The theory–practice gap in nurse education: its cases and possible solutions. *Journal of Advanced Nursing* **16**: 1055–61.

Maslach, C. 1981 *Burnout: the Cost of Caring*. New Jersey: Prentice-Hall.

Meerabeau, L. 1992 Tacit nursing knowledge: an untapped resource or a methodological headache? *Journal of Advanced Nursing* **17**: 108–12.

Melia, K.M. 1987 *Learning and Working: the Occupational Socialisation of Nurses*. London: Tavistock.

Menzies, I.E.P. 1959 The functioning of social systems as a defence against anxiety – a report on a study of the nursing service within a general hospital. *Human Relations* **13**: 95–121.

Meyer, J. 1993 New paradigm research in practice: the trials and tribulations of action research. *Journal of Advanced Nursing* **18**: 1066–72.

Obholzer, A. and Roberts, V.Z. 1994 *The Unconscious at Work. Individual and Organisational Stress in the Human Services*. London: Routledge.

O'Callagahan, J. and Cowie, H. 1995 Video in counselling training – an exploratory study. *Therapist* **3**: 29–32.

Parry, E. and Richardson, A. 1996 *NHS Psychotherapy Services in England. Review of Strategic Policy*. NHS Executive: Department of Health.

Peplau, H.E. 1952 *Interpersonal Relations in Nursing*. New York: Putnam.

Platt-Koch, L.M. 1986 Clinical supervision for psychiatric nurses. *Journal of Psychosocial Nursing* **26**: 7–15.

Polanyi, M. 1967 *The Tacit Dimension*. London: Routledge.

Powell, J.H. 1989 The reflective practitioner in nursing. *Journal of Advanced Nursing* **14**: 824–32.

Proctor, B. 1986 Supervision: a co-operative exercise in accountability. In: Marken, M. and Payne, M. (eds) *Enabling and Insuring: Supervision in Practice*. Leicester: National Youth Bureau and Council for Education and Training in Youth and Community Work.

Rafferty, M. and Coleman, M. 1995 Educating nurses to understand clinical supervision in practice. *Nursing Standard* **10**(45): 38–41.

Savage, J. 1990 The theory and practice of new nursing. *Nursing Times* **86**(4): 42–5.

Saylor, C.R. 1990 Reflection and professional education: art, science and competency. *Nurse Educator* **15**: 8–11.

Scanlon, C. and Baillie, A.P. 1994 'A preparation for practice?' Students' experiences of counselling training within departments of higher education. *Counselling Psychology Quarterly* **7**: 407–27.

Schon, D.A. 1983 *The Reflective Practitioner*. New York: Basic Books.

Schon, D.A. 1987 *Educating the Reflective Practitioner*. London: Jossey Bass.

Sharpe, M. 1994 *The Third Eye. Supervision of Analytic Groups*. London: Routledge.

Sharpe, M. 1995 Training of supervisors. In: Sharpe, M. (ed.) *The Third Eye. Supervision of Analytic Groups*. London: Routledge.

Skynner, A.C.R. 1989 *Institutes and How to Survive Them: Mental Health Training and Consultation*. London: Routledge.

Stockwell, E. 1972 *The Unpopular Patient*. London: Royal College of Nursing.

Travelbee, J. 1971 *Intervention in Psychiatric Nursing. Process in the One to One Relationship*. Philadelphia: FA Davis.

UKCC (United Kingdom Central Council for Nurses and Midwives) 1996 *A Position Statement on Clinical Supervision for Nursing and Health Visiting*. London: UKCC.

Wright, H. 1989 *Groupwork: Perspectives and Practice*. London: Scutari Press.

Wright, H. 1991 The patient, the nurse, his life and her mother: psychodynamic influences in nursing education and practice. *Psychoanalytic Psychotherapy* 5(2): 139–49.

Wright, S.G. 1992 Modelling excellence: the role of the consultant nurse. In: Butterworth, T. and Faugier, J. (eds) *Clinical Supervision and Mentorship in Nursing*. London: Chapman & Hall.

8

Instruments for Evaluating Clinical Supervision

Jerome Carson

Despite the clear importance attached to clinical supervision across all professional groups, the actual process of supervision remains surprisingly poorly evaluated. Nursing is no exception to this rule. In this chapter, I stress the need to develop measures to evaluate supervision that are based on the principles of reliability, validity and utility. Five scales that have been used in the Clinical Supervision Evaluation Project are described in detail: the general health questionnaire (GHQ–28), the Maslach burnout inventory, the Minnesota job satisfaction scale, the Cooper coping skills scale and the nurse stress index. In addition to the use of quantitative methods, qualitative approaches also have an important role to play, especially in illustrating the 'lived experience' of supervision. As so little research has been conducted to date, much evaluative work remains to be done. One priority is the need to develop a questionnaire measure of the supervision process. Researchers also need to demonstrate how the provision of clinical supervision for staff can lead to improved patient outcomes.

Introduction

Research in supervision is the biggest joke in our profession. There is no distinct body of knowledge to uncover. (Holloway, 1995, p. xi)

Supervision is an assumed rather than proven educational benefit. There are plenty of published articles of a theoretical or anecdotal nature, but precious few that have conducted any empirical investigation of the supervisory process and its outcomes. (Green, 1995, p. 41)

While the first quotation is taken from the field of counselling and the second from clinical psychology, both could equally have been drawn from nursing. It is generally assumed that clinical supervision is a beneficial process. The above statements imply that this may be more myth than fact. In this chapter, I start off by briefly examining clinical supervision in nursing. I consider a range of approaches to evaluating clinical supervision in nursing and then outline key principles that should guide our use of rating scales as evaluation instruments. Finally, I examine five measures that may usefully be employed to evaluate clinical supervision.

Clinical supervision in nursing

The UKCC, in its position statement on clinical supervision (UKCC, 1996), stated that 'evaluation of clinical supervision is needed to assess how it influences care, practice standards and the service. Evaluation systems should be determined locally' (key statement 6). The statement went on to make the point made earlier that there is a lack of information on the benefits and outcomes of clinical supervision. However, as several other chapters in this book deal with the issue of supervision in nursing, I will touch on it only briefly. Simms (1993) stated that 'there is a growing and acknowledged awareness of and commitment to the value of supervision and the supervisor relationship'. Yet she conceded that there is 'very little published research' (p. 328). Faugier (1996, p. 53) reports that 'Until recently little of any substance had been published in the nursing literature, and the absence of empirical data on clinical supervision remains widespread in all fields, particularly in nursing'.

A typical nursing research study on clinical supervision is that published by Ritter *et al.* (1996). In this paper, they describe the supervision framework that they have developed for general nursing students undertaking clinical experience in psychiatric wards. They provide much helpful detail about the methods they use with students, such as critical incident analysis, life charts and genograms. However, they provide no data on how students perceive these experiences. Is their method better for students than the previous methods adopted? Are there particular aspects of the supervisory experience that students value and learn from more than others? So while Ritter *et al.* have provided a helpful account of their methods, they provide no data whatsoever on its evaluation.

Similarly, Faugier (1996) has provided a helpful model of the key requirements of positive supervisory experiences. She suggests that supervisors need to be generous, rewarding, open, willing to learn, thoughtful and thought provoking, humane, sensitive, uncompromising in standards, adaptable and practice focused, to provide a safe relationship and to establish trust. Apart from providing an example of the model in action (Butterworth and Faugier, 1992), there is no empirical evidence to substantiate this model, appealing though it seems.

One of the most influential models is that of Proctor (1986). Proctor conceives of clinical supervision as fulfilling three main functions: normative, formative and restorative. The normative or managerial aspects of supervision imply an aspect of overseeing and monitoring standards. This involves caseload management, making the supervisee aware of organisational policies and procedures, and checking record-keeping. Butterworth (1996) suggests that it could be evaluated by audits of clinical supervision, by looking at sickness and absence rates, and by surveys of job satisfaction.

Restorative or supportive aspects of clinical supervision are concerned with the creation of a supervisory relationship in which the supervisee feels valued and understood. It involves recognition of the stresses inherent in the nursing role. This can be monitored by measures such as the Maslach burnout scale (Maslach and Jackson, 1986), which examines the degree to which nurses are emotionally affected by their work.

The third element is the formative or educational component. This is concerned with the identification and development of skills in supervisees and the integration of theory with practice. Butterworth (1996) suggests a number of ways in which the formative component can be evaluated. He recommends Trust-wide educational audits to check that staff are still involving themselves in continuing education. He also mentions the use of IPR and states that sessions with clients could be taped using either video or audio formats, to enable supervisors to monitor the development of supervisees' therapeutic skills.

Approaches to evaluating clinical supervision

The simple use of quantitative measures to evaluate the complex process of clinical supervision is no guarantee of accuracy. During my own training as a clinical psychologist, we were, at the end of each clinical placement, rated on a number of key competencies, such as report-writing. The rating scale used had a number of categories: Excellent, Very good, Better than average, Average, Below average and Fail. An analysis of ratings for all trainees across all placements showed that almost 90 per cent of trainees were at least better than average.

Perhaps in light of such experience, the largest clinical psychology training course at University College London has moved towards a totally qualitative form of assessment. Their form assesses 14 specific competencies, such as professional behaviour, relationship with colleagues and interviewing skills. Supervisors are asked to rate the supervisee on their 'Use of supervision'. The guidelines provided for raters are as follows: 'Uses supervision flexibly to meet training needs, i.e. to seek reassurance, anxiety reduction, to gain feedback or to learn, as appropriate. Asks for advice and guidance and is receptive to feedback. Or, needs to learn better use of supervision, e.g. has a poor response to constructive criticism, does not ask for feedback, seems not to listen to or act on advice.' Supervisors are then expected to add their interpretation of the supervisee's performance during supervision sessions below these guidelines. Interestingly, supervisees also get a chance to rate supervisors on the quality of their supervision, for example, 'Supervision arrangements' – amount, reliability, availability, approachability. They are also asked to comment on whether supervision has been facilitative in a separate section. Such approaches are purely qualitative in nature but may be much better at capturing the dynamic nature of the supervisory relationship. It is fair to say that mechanisms for assessing student performance in supervision are much more clearly and carefully worked out than are mechanisms for evaluating post-qualification supervision.

There is a clear need empirically to evaluate clinical supervision in nursing and other disciplines. The Manchester University clinical supervision evaluation project, described elsewhere in this book, marks a major step in evaluating clinical supervision in 23 separate centres. The measures used in the project are described later in this chapter. There is, however, a need for second-generation studies that take this work a stage further. For example, if we could reliably rate supervisors on Faugier's 13 key requirements for positive supervision, we could then examine the learning outcomes for students with facilitative supervisors against those with less open attitudes. We might expect that students of facilitative supervisors have more positive mental health outcomes, for example are less burned out, than do supervisees with more difficult supervisors. It would be important to supplement this information with in-depth interviews. What were critical incidents in supervision? What did supervisees find helpful/ unhelpful? It would be important to try to obtain this information when supervisees are on placement rather than retrospectively.

Principles guiding the selection of measures

Streiner (1993a) provides a helpful checklist for evaluating the content of rating scales. The first issue he considers is the selection of *items*. Where do items in scales come from? He makes the interesting observation that 'borrowing from one source is plagiarism, but taking from two or more is research' (p. 141). Items for scales are generally taken from previous scales, clinical observation, expert opinion, patients' reports or theory. Once items have been selected for any scale, it is important that detailed item analysis is then conducted. This examines issues such as endorsement frequency or, more simply, how often people answer particular questions. One of the purposes of any questionnaire is to be able to discriminate between groups of people who complete it. If 99 per cent of respondents answered a particular item, it would not be very discriminating. Similarly, restrictions in the range of responses are also important to avoid. We can assess this by looking at the frequency of responses to each item. What we want to aim for is a good distribution of responses. If we are using a five-point scale with an undecided category in the middle, and the majority of respondents select this response, it adds little to our questionnaire. It is important to assess comprehension: what may seem a reasonable item to us may not be understandable to some respondents. Some items may have ambiguous meaning. We need also to ensure that items do not have value-laden or offensive content. Rust and Golombok (1989) give a practical example of how to construct a new questionnaire.

Another issue to consider is item discrimination analysis. Given the point made earlier that the main purpose of questionnaires is to discriminate between populations, it is helpful to include items that discriminate between high and low scorers. This is done by looking at the individual responses to every item for high and low scorers. For some items, there will be differences between both groups in how they respond to the item; these are the items we wish to keep in the scale. Finally, we will want to consider the correlations of each item with total scores. Correlations range from +1.0 to –1.0. They are measured using statistical tests such as Pearson's product moment correlation coefficient or Spearman's rho. If an item does not, on one of these tests, correlate more than 0.2 with total score, it may be assessing something completely different. Likewise, if several items intercorrelate highly with each other, there may be some item redundancy. We may then be able to cut down the number of items. A paper by our own research group (Brown *et al.*, 1995) illustrates several of these points.

The second issue to consider is *reliability*. In essence, reliability is to do with the accuracy of a measure. If we have a scale that measures anxiety, its reliability is to do with how accurately it measures anxiety. Reliability is assessed in a number of ways. Internal consistency is to do with how consistently the individual scores on items assessing the same phenomenon. If there are 10 questions that assess anxiety, we can compare the individual's scores on the first five items against their scores on the last five (split-half reliability). Alternatively, we can compare their scores on odd-numbered items 1, 3, 5, 7, 9 against their scores for items 2, 4, 6, 8, 10 (odd–even reliability). The most widely used method for assessing internal reliability is Cronbach's alpha (Cronbach, 1951). Fortunately, modern computer-based statistical packages such as SPSS for Windows (Norussis, 1993; Kinnear and Gray, 1994) make the process of estimating scale reliability a relatively simple business.

It is also important to know about the test–retest reliability of rating scales. If we administer a depression scale to individuals, and then reassess them on the same scale 2 weeks later, assuming of course that nothing major has happened in their lives in the intervening period, their scores on the two occasions should be quite similar.

With behaviour rating scales, it is also important to consider inter-rater agreement. Do both raters see the patient similarly? Good scales have high reliability, reported as correlation coefficients of more than 0.70.

Validity is the third issue to explore. Put simply, the validity of any scale is whether it measures what it purports to. Like reliability, it is assessed in a variety of ways. Face validity asks this simple question: do the items appear, on the face of it, to measure what they are trying to.

Content validity is a more systematic assessment of whether the scale contains the most relevant aspects of the construct. A scale for depression needs to cover both biological aspects of depression, such as weight loss, sleep disturbance and loss of libido, and psychological aspects, such as pessimism and hopelessness. Criterion validity comprises both concurrent and predictive validity. Concurrent criterion validity assesses the degree to which a scale correlates with existing measures of the same phenomenon. Predictive validity occurs when a person's test score is used to make predictions about his or her future behaviour. For example, staff who score high on stress scales are likely to take more time off sick in the following 6 months than are staff low on stress.

Finally, construct validity is to do with the accumulation of research evidence that is built up over time with respect or a particular construct. For instance, Eysenck (1980) has conducted a whole range of studies that link the phenomena of extroversion and introversion with biological factors such as conditionability and then links this to criminality and neuroticism. Extroversion can be reliably assessed using the 90-item Eysenck personality questionnaire (Eysenck and Eysenck, 1975).

Before leaving the concepts of reliability and validity, it is important to note on which specific client populations these have been assessed. It used to be somewhat disparagingly said that American psychology was the psychology of the American undergraduate student as many of the classic studies in the field had been conducted on students. Indeed, students in America are given course credits for participating as volunteers in research studies. It is important for clinical scales to be piloted on established clinical populations rather than on students, who are not typical of the wider population.

The final issue to consider is *utility*. How long does it take to complete a measure? How much training is needed to administer the scale? Finally, is the scale easy to score and interpret? Related to this, we have to consider how accessible the scale is and, for published scales, how much they cost to purchase. Readers who wish to learn more about scale construction should refer to Streiner and Norman (1989). Streiner has also written a number of user-friendly accounts of other aspects of research methodology in a series of papers in the *Canadian Journal of Psychiatry* (see Streiner, 1990, 1993b, 1994, 1995, 1996a, b; Goering and Streiner, 1996).

Selected instruments for evaluating clinical supervision

There are literally hundreds of questionnaires that could be suitable for evaluating clinical supervision. In this section, I restrict the choice to only five. There are two main reasons for this. First, we used only five questionnaires plus a demographic measure in the Clinical Supervision Evaluation Project (Butterworth *et al.*, 1996). Second, space allows me only to give a brief introduction to the range of measures, so those chosen have well-established reliability and validity.

Nurse stress index

This is a 30-item measure of nursing stress (Harris *et al.*, 1988). Harris (1989) describes the development of the scale. Nurses are asked to rate how much pressure each of the 30 items has caused them in the past 3 months. Scores range from 'causes me no pressure' =1, to 'causes me extreme pressure' =5. The questionnaire has six subscales. These are Managing the Workload 1 (sample item: 'Trivial tasks interfere with my professional role'), Managing the Workload 2 (sample: 'My nursing and administrative roles conflict'), Organisational Support and Involvement (sample: 'I only get feedback when my performance is unsatisfactory'), Dealing with Patients and Relatives (sample: 'Difficulty in dealing with aggressive people'), Home Work Conflict (sample: 'Job versus home demands'), and Confidence and Competence in Role (sample: 'Lack of specialised training for specialised task'). Unlike other measures of nursing staff stress, such as the nurse stress scale (Grey-Toft and Anderson, 1981a, b), the nurse stress index has been developed in Britain. In addition to scores on the six subscales mentioned above, a total stress score is also obtained.

A number of the items in this scale are closely linked to issues that might be raised in clinical supervision settings. It is therefore a helpful scale to evaluate the supervision process. As it was developed in close consultation with many nurses from several centres, it has very good content validity. The authors present evidence for the scale's concurrent validity by comparing it with the Crown Crisp experiential index (Crown and Crisp, 1979). The scale also has good reliability.

Maslach burnout inventory

This scale is probably the most widely used measure in nursing stress studies worldwide. Developed by Maslach and Jackson (1986), it has 22 items that cover the three independent dimensions of occupational burnout syndrome. Respondents are asked how often they experience the characteristics of burnout on a scale from 0 = 'never', to 6 = 'every day'. Emotional Exhaustion has nine items, such as 'I feel emotionally drained from my work'. The second dimension, Depersonalisation, has five items, for example 'I feel I treat some recipients (patients) as if they were impersonal objects'. The third dimension, Personal Accomplishment, has eight items, including 'I feel I have accomplished many worthwhile things in this job'. Apart from obtaining scores on each dimension, scores can also be converted into a categorical score, i.e. whether a person has high, moderate or low burnout on a particular dimension. Recent reviews of the scale have been provided by Schaufeli *et al.* (1993) and Leiter and Harvie (1996). In terms of its reliability, the Maslach scale has both high internal consistency and high test–retest reliability. Its validity has also been well established (Sandoval, 1989).

The Maslach scale does not specifically address issues of clinical supervision. However, we might expect nurses who are well supervised and supported to have lower occupational burnout than nurses without such support. The strength of the scale is that it can help to assess the *restorative* aspects of clinical supervision.

General health questionnaire

There are four versions of this particular scale, which refer to the number of items they contain, hence GHQ–12, GHQ–28, GHQ–30 and GHQ–60 (Goldberg and Williams, 1988). The scale measures an individual's level of psychological distress. Apart from providing an overall GHQ score, cut-offs are said to discriminate between those individuals who might be regarded as 'psychiatric cases' on the basis of their scores. On the GHQ–28, the cut-off for psychiatric 'caseness' is a score of 5 or more. Using this criterion, some 41 per cent of community mental health nurses in the large Claybury study would be classified as 'cases', (Carson *et al.*, 1995). High as this might seem, it is lower than the figures for social work students of 62 per cent and for postgraduate certificate of education students of 91 per cent reported by Tobin and Carson (1994). This scale is now the most widely used psychiatric screening tool worldwide (Bowling, 1995). As one might expect with such a popular scale, its psychometric properties have been well established. Split-half and test–retest reliability coefficients are high. The scale has good content, criterion and construct validity.

The 28-item format has four sections with seven questions each. Somatic Symptoms asks about distressing bodily symptoms such as 'Felt that you were ill'. This is rated as 'not at all', 'no more than usual', 'rather more than usual' and 'much more than usual'. Using the GHQ scoring method, the individual scores a point only for either of the last two responses. The other sections are Anxiety and Insomnia (e.g. 'Lost much sleep over worry'), Social Role Functioning (e.g. 'Been taking longer over the things that you do') and Severe Depression (e.g. 'Felt that life isn't worth living'). Again, as with the burnout scale, the GHQ does not directly assess clinical supervision; however, it again enables us to assess the restorative component.

Cooper coping skills scale

This is another 28-item scale that is used to assess the frequency with which individuals utilise particular coping strategies. A six-point scale is used to denote how often a strategy is used, from 1 = 'never used by me', to 6 = 'very extensively used by me'. The scale has six subscales (Cooper *et al.*, 1988). These are Social Support – four items (e.g. 'Talk to understanding friends'), Task Strategies – seven items (e.g. 'Plan ahead'), Logic – three items (e.g. 'Try to stand aside and think through the situation'), Time – four items (e.g. 'Deal with the problems immediately as they occur'), and Involvement – six items (e.g. 'Look for ways to make the work more interesting'). Scores are obtained for each subscale. Independent researchers have, however, found that the best single measure of a person's coping skills is the total coping skills score, rather than any of the single subscales (Broers *et al.*, 1995; Kirkcaldy *et al.*, 1995). Work conducted by our own research team demon-strates that nursing staff who utilise many coping skills experience significantly less psychological distress on the GHQ–28, as well as lower emotional exhaustion on the Maslach scale, than nurses who use few coping skills. Furthermore, high coping skills staff take less time off sick (Carson *et al.*, 1996). The internal consistency of this scale is quite variable, and further work is needed on its psychometric properties. While coping skills do not relate directly to clinical supervision, they are nonetheless very important moderators of stress (Fagin *et al.*, 1996).

Minnesota job satisfaction scale

A final instrument to consider in helping to evaluate clinical supervision is this 20-item questionnaire, developed at the University of Minnesota by Weiss and his colleagues (Weiss *et al.*, 1967) and based on Herzberg's theory of work motivation. Items are rated on a five-point scale from 1 = 'very dissatisfied', to 5 = 'very satisfied'. Three separate scores are obtained. Intrinsic Satisfaction (12 items) reflects a person's degree of contentment with the job itself in terms of achievement, recognition or responsibility. Extrinsic Satisfaction (six items) looks at contentment with factors such as salary, status, security and supervision (e.g. 'The competence of my supervisor in making decisions'). Both scores are combined, along with two additional items, to give a total job satisfaction score. The reliability and validity of the scale has been established with nurses both in America (Koelbel *et al.*, 1991) and in Britain (Waite *et al.*, 1996). Job satisfaction is clearly a very important factor in all jobs. Staff who are satisfied in their work are more likely to deliver better standards of patient care.

Conclusion

Most health care professionals are aware of the importance of clinical supervision, and all professional bodies regard clinical supervision as critical to the development of skills in supervisees to ensure that practitioners maintain a high standard of care. Despite the clear importance given to clinical supervision, it has received surprisingly little attention from researchers.

In this chapter, I have outlined the key principles that should guide evaluation efforts. This includes careful questionnaire construction with close attention to issues of reliability, validity and utility. I have described five scientifically validated measures that could be used to evaluate clinical supervision. Any comprehensive evaluation will need to encompass quantitative and qualitative methodologies. Quantitative measures enable comparison across studies, whereas qualitative methods describe the 'lived experience' of clinical supervision. Systematic evaluation of clinical supervision will enable us to move towards a better understanding of the dynamic process of supervision. Ultimately, this has the potential to lead to better patient care.

Appendix

The nurse stress index is available from: Resource Assessment and Development, Claro Court, Claro Road, Harrogate, North Yorkshire HG1 4BA. Tel: (01423) 529529. Fax: (01423) 508005.

The Maslach burnout inventory can be obtained from: Oxford Psychologists, Lambourne House, 311–321 Banbury Road, Oxford OX2 7JH. Tel: (01865) 510203. Fax: (01865) 310368.

The general health questionnaire is supplied by: NFER-Nelson, Darville House, 2 Oxford Road East, Windsor, Berkshire SL4 1DF. Tel: (01753) 858961. Fax: (01753) 856830.

The Cooper coping skills scale is also obtainable from NFER-Nelson. It is a part of the occupational stress indicator, and special permission may be needed to use it separately.

The Minnesota job satisfaction scale is now probably out of print. Readers interested in obtaining a copy should write to me at the Institute of Psychiatry in London.

References

Bowling, A. 1995 *Measuring Disease*. Buckingham: Open University Press.
Broers, P., Evers, A. and Cooper, C. 1995 Differences in occupational stress in three European countries. *International Journal of Stress Management* **2**(4): 171–80.
Brown, D., Leary, J., Carson, J., Bartlett, H. and Fagin, L. 1995 Stress and the community mental health nurse: the development of a measure. *Journal of Psychiatric and Mental Health Nursing* **2**(1): 9–12.

Butterworth, T. 1996 Primary attempts at research based evaluation of clinical supervision. *NT Research* **1**(2): 96–101.

Butterworth T. and Faugier, J. 1992 Supervision for life. In: Butterworth, T. and Faugier, J. (eds) *Clinical Supervision and Mentorship in Nursing*. London: Chapman & Hall.

Butterworth, T., Bishop, V. and Carson, J. 1996 First steps towards
evaluating clinical supervision in nursing and health visiting. Part
1: Theory, policy and practice development. A review. *Journal
of Clinical Nursing* **5**(1): 25–35.

Carson, J., Cooper, C., Fagin, L. *et al.* 1996 Coping skills in mental
health nursing: do they make a difference? *Journal of Psychiatric
and Mental Health Nursing* **3**(3): 201–2.

Carson, J., Fagin, L. and Ritter, S. (eds) 1995 *Stress and Coping in
Mental Health Nursing*. London: Chapman & Hall.

Cooper, C., Sloan, S. and Williams, S. 1988 *The Occupational Stress
Indicator*. Windsor: NFER-Nelson.

Cronbach, L. 1951 Coefficient alpha and the internal structure of
tests. *Psychometrika* **16**: 297–334.

Crown, S. and Crisp, A. 1979 *Manual of the Crown–Crisp Experiential Index*. London: Hodder & Stoughton.

Eysenck, H. 1980 The bio-social model of man and the unifica-
tion of psychology. In: Chapman, A. and Jones, D. (eds) *Models
of Man*. Leicester: British Psychological Society.

Eysenck, H. and Eysenck, S. 1975 *Manual for the Eysenck Personality Questionnaire*. London: Hodder & Stoughton.

Fagin, L., Carson, J., Leary, J. *et al.* 1996 Stress, coping and burnout
in mental health nurses: findings from three research studies.
International Journal of Social Psychiatry **42**(2): 102–11.

Faugier, J. 1996 Clinical supervision and mental health nursing.
In: Sandford, T. and Gournay, K. (eds) *Perspectives in Mental
Health Nursing*. London: Baillière Tindall.

Goering, P. and Streiner, D. 1996 Reconcilable differences: the
marriage of qualitative and quantitative methods. *Canadian
Journal of Psychiatry* **41**(8): 491–7.

Goldberg, D. and Williams, S. 1988 *A User's Guide to the General
Health Questionnaire*. Windsor: NFER-Nelson.

Green, D. 1995 Supervision for qualified clinical psychologists. *Clinical Psychology Forum* **80**: 40–1.

Grey-Toft, P. and Anderson, J. 1981a The Nursing Stress Scale:
the development of an instrument. *Journal of Behavioural Assessment* **3**: 11–23.

Grey-Toft, P. and Anderson, J. 1981b Stress amongst hospital
nursing staff: its causes and effects. *Social Science and Medicine*
15: 639–47.

Harris, P. 1989 The Nurse Stress Index. *Work and Stress* **5**(4): 335–46.
Harris, P., Hingley, P. and Cooper, C. 1988 *The Nurse Stress Index User's Guide*. Harrogate: Resource Assessment and Development.
Holloway, E. 1995 *Clinical Supervision: A Systems Approach*. California: Sage.
Kinnear, P. and Gray, C. 1994 *SPSS for Windows Made Simple*. Hove: Lawrence Erlbaum.
Kirkcaldy, B., Cooper, C. and Brown, J. 1995 The role of coping in the stress–strain relationship among senior police officers. *International Journal of Stress Management* **2**(2): 69–78.
Koelbel, P., Fuller, F. and Misener, T. 1991 Job satisfaction of nurse practitioners: an analysis using Herzberg's theory. *Nurse Practitioner* **16**(4): 43–6.
Leiter, M. and Harvie, P. 1996 Burnout among mental health workers: a review and a research agenda. *International Journal of Social Psychiatry* **42**(4): 90–101.
Maslach, C. and Jackson, S. 1986 *Maslach Burnout Inventory*. California: Consulting Psychologists Press.
Norussis, M. 1993 *SPSS for Windows: Base System User's Guide*. Chicago, Il: SPSS Inc.
Proctor, B. 1986 Supervision: a co-operative exercise in accountability. In: Marken, A. and Payne, M. (eds) *Enabling and Ensuring: Supervision in Practice*. Leicester: National Youth Bureau.
Ritter, S., Norman, I., Rentoul, L. and Bodley, D. 1996 A model of clinical supervision for nurses undertaking short placements in mental health care settings. *Journal of Clinical Nursing* **5**: 149–58.
Rust, J. and Golombok, S. 1989 *Modern Psychometrics: The Science of Psychological Assessment*. London: Routledge.
Sandoval, J. 1989 Review of the Maslach Burnout Inventory. In: Close-Caroly, K. and Kramer, J. (eds) *Mental Measurement Yearbook 10*. Lincoln, Neb.: Buros Institute of Mental Measurement.
Schaufeli, W., Maslach, C. and Marek, T. 1993 *Professional Burnout: Recent Developments in Theory and Practice*. Washington: Taylor & Francis.
Simms, J. 1993 Supervision. In: Wright, H. and Giddey, M. (eds) *Mental Health Nursing: From First Principles to Professional Practice*. London: Chapman & Hall.
Streiner, D. 1990 Sample size and power in psychiatric research. *Canadian Journal of Psychiatry* **35**(7): 616–20.
Streiner, D. 1993a A checklist for evaluating the usefulness of rating scales. *Canadian Journal of Psychiatry* **38**(2): 140–8.
Streiner, D. 1993b An introduction to multivariate statistics. *Canadian Journal of Psychiatry* **38**(2): 140–8.

Streiner, D. 1994 Figuring out factors: the use and misuse of factor analysis. *Canadian Journal of Psychiatry* **39**(3): 135–40.

Streiner, D. 1995 Learning how to differ: agreement and reliability statistics in psychiatry. *Canadian Journal of Psychiatry* **40**(2): 60–6.

Streiner, D. 1996a While you're up get me a grant. A guide to grant writing. *Canadian Journal of Psychiatry* **41**(3):137–43.

Streiner, D. 1996b Maintaining standards: differences between the standard deviation and standard error, and how to use each. *Canadian Journal of Psychiatry* **41**(8): 498–501.

Streiner, D. and Norman, G. 1989 *Health Measurement Scales: A Practical Guide to their Development and Use*. Oxford: Oxford University Press.

Tobin, P.J. and Carson, J. 1994 Stress and the student social worker: a preliminary investigation. *Social Work and Social Sciences Review* **5**(3): 246–55.

Waite, A., Oliver, N., Carson, J. and Fagin, L. 1996 Mental health nursing: is community or ward based nursing more satisfying?. *Psychiatric Care* **2**(5): 167–70.

Weiss, D., Dawis, R., England, G. and Lofquist, L. 1967 *Manual for the Minnesota Satisfaction Questionnaire*. University of Minnesota: Industrial Relations Centre.

UKCC (United Kingdom Central Council for Nursing, Midwifery and Health Visiting) 1966 *Position Statement on Clinical Supervision for Nursing, Midwifery and Health Visiting*. London: UKCC.

9

The Potential of Clinical Supervision for Nurses, Midwives and Health Visitors

Anthony Butterworth

This chapter provides a short review of matters of importance in the development of clinical supervision over the preceding decade. Arguments are made that support from policy-makers and professional bodies is important in moving forward with clinical supervision and that the demand to link all professional developments to positive patient outcome is both necessary and probably impossible. Safe and accountable practice is vitally important, and clinical supervision is providing support to both safety and accountability.

Introduction

From tentative beginnings 10 years ago, the implementation of clinical supervision and the debate that surrounds it appears to have reached a peak. Can the momentum in its development be sustained? Is there sufficient academic strength and practical utility in clinical supervision to offer advantage to both the profession and the patients and families they care for?

Clinical supervision certainly appears to have won the hearts of those who occupy both ends of the spectrum between the humanistic phenomenologists and the problem-focused behaviouralists characteristic of British nursing. Nursing itself has undergone striking changes in the past decade. New roles and structures and demands for advanced practice have asked great things of nurses. Exciting times indeed, but the need to surround these new ways of working with safe supportive supervision and debate is equally as important.

There are tensions which have yet to be resolved, not least of which is the very title 'clinical supervision'. There are those who take exception to the term 'clinical supervision', indeed, the UKCC has extensively debated the point is its run-up to a final statement (UKCC, 1996). I believe that a confident, expert professional has little to fear from being supervised. If the concern of clinical supervision is to sustain and develop professional practice, its intentions are clearly honourable and not to be feared. Doubts about being supervised most often relate to supervision's potential to be abused as a system of unnecessary control and interference in professional autonomy. Putting to one side the debate about how much autonomy we think we have, these fears are not unreasonable, especially given the management styles in some Trusts. In greater part, however, I believe that clinical supervision is a practice-led activity and, when secured within this practice embrace, is less likely to be abused.

There is growing evidence that other professions are beginning to explore the ideas surrounding clinical supervision. Managers, senior medical staff and general practitioners are experimenting with what they call (somewhat confusingly for nurses) mentorship schemes. These schemes show some of the characteristics of clinical supervision, and there are points at which these matters can be explored through multidisciplinary work.

An important debate lies in attempting to make judgements on the impact that clinical supervision has on patients and their families. Attempts are being made (more often through argument than action) to relate the impact of clinical supervision to patient outcome. These arguments at worst prevent services implementing clinical supervision or spending time and money investing in it, and at best suggest that, while the importance of impacting on patient outcome is undeniable, absolutely everything else, including the health and well-being of the workforce, is subsumed by it.

These attempts to link clinical supervision to patient outcome are not well advanced and may indeed prove so elusive and complex to construct in real life that no-one will attempt them. At present, what is more easy to demonstrate is the link between clinical supervision, work practices and the well-being of the workforce. This is in itself a worthy endeavour, and its value should not be underestimated.

Clinical supervision: what is it?

Has progress been made on assessing the utility of theoretical models and clinical supervision? The appropriateness of a number of theoretical models has caused some debate but there is room for substantially more. Assertions that it was some kind of counselling, that clinical supervision was well established in mental health nursing or that midwives had been doing it for years have been to some extent unmasked as the wider implications of clinical supervision have been recognised. A realisation that the psychodynamic models often adopted by mental health nurses (Mahmood, 1994) or the organisational/structural models of midwifery (Harris, 1994) may be inappropriate for nurses in acute surgery or intensive care has dawned, and there is a need to develop models that best serve a particular specialty and locality. In the proper search for appropriate models, it will be tragic if the generous and central intentions of clinical supervision for the support of practice delivered at the highest quality are lost as self-indulgent theoreticians develop and promote models that have less to do with utility and more to do with having a particular 'species' named after oneself. Encouragingly, most developments in clinical supervision are being led by those with immediate practice experience, so the issue of theory being dislocated from practice may not be quite as problematic.

There appears to be an acceptance that the composite elements offered by Proctor (1991) have found favour among the profession. Her description of the normative (organisational responsibility), formative (development of skills) and restorative (supporting personal well-being) as the key elements of clinical supervision are popular.

The delivery of clinical supervision, frequently based around ideas suggested by Houston (1990), has had a fairly general acceptance. One-to-one sessions with a supervisor from the same discipline have been reported (Dewing, 1994), as has one-to-one peer supervision (Semperingham, 1994). Peer group supervision has found favour particularly among district nurses and health visitors (Johnson, 1995), and networking supervision is reportedly used by nurse specialists in such areas as HIV/AIDS care and Macmillan nursing, reports from this appearing soon (Jones, 1997). The cost consequences of implementing clinical supervision may hinder its implementation, but such little evidence as there is shows the consequences to be under-researched (Dudley and Butterworth, 1994).

Brocklehurst (1995), in his debate on the emerging literature, suggests a shift in definition from one in which clinical supervision is 'an enabling relationship between nurses whereby one nurse is accountable to another nurse in helping them practice to the best of their ability' (Butterworth, 1988) to one in which there is 'an exchange between practising professionals to enable the development of professional skills' (Butterworth, 1992). This may be evidence of sensitivity to the practical and political difficulties of delivering clinical supervision and the cost consequences associated with it. The debate will inevitably benefit as further changes are identified in the gathering and reporting of data.

The international literature demonstrates some discussion by nurses in other countries on the subject of clinical supervision. Definitions inevitably have different meanings because of the sociocultural influences of each nation, but some general observations are possible. The literature talks widely of 'supervisors' in the USA. The meaning is particular and refers most often to a 'superior/novitiate' type of relationship that has a strong management focus. The term 'clinical supervision' is sometimes used as a term of reference for supervisors, although the interpretation has no apparent difference. There have been more generous interpretations by authors seeking to develop clinical supervision to gather in personal and professional development (Platt-Koch, 1986), although this type of discussion is less common. Thought-provoking debates have arisen in such areas as mentorship and preceptorship (Darling, 1985) with interesting titles such as 'What to do about toxic mentors'; these carry lessons of common interest to all those working in clinical supervision. Japanese nurses appear to have taken on American models (Ito, 1984). German nurses report a view of clinical supervision that is more growth-promoting and developmental (Olbrich, 1985), while Australian nurses are beginning to raise the subject through conference agendas (P. Armitage, personal communication, 1995). In Scandinavia, research has progressed to examine the impact of clinical supervision on nurses working with patients with dementia (Hallberg and Norberg, 1993). The authors go so far as to suggest that interventions with patients are improved by the use of clinical supervision.

Relationship between policy and practice

There is little doubt that health care policy has had considerable influence on the development of clinical supervision in the UK. What may essentially begin as good ideas in professional development may not progress if not underwritten by policy influence or support from the DoH. The introduction of the *Code of Professional Conduct* (UKCC, 1984) and *The Scope of Professional Practice* (UKCC, 1992) has significance when considering autonomy and accountability in practice within the reduced professional support mechanisms in flattened hierarchies. Clinical supervision has been seen to provide a useful framework for the DoH for developing and supporting those in practice and has consequently received the support of strategic planning from the Chief Nursing Officer (CNO) and others. The CNO recommended in the policy plan *Vision for the Future* (DoH, 1993) that 'the concept of clinical supervision should be further explored and developed. Discussions should be held at a local and national level on the range and appropriateness of models of clinical supervision and a report made available to the professions'.

This report, *Clinical Supervision: A Position Paper* (Faugier and Butterworth, 1994), was produced the following year and widely distributed to the profession by the DoH. In an accompanying letter, the CNO stated, 'I have no doubt as to the value of clinical supervision and consider it to be fundamental to safeguarding standards, the development of professional expertise and the delivery of care' (DoH, 1994a). The recent Allitt enquiry (1991) has also crystallised a number of concerns about the supervision of safe and accountable practice. It has been argued that clinical supervision can help to sustain and develop safe and accountable practice (Butterworth and Faugier, 1992). It has also been commonly agreed and endorsed by participants in a Delphi survey of optimum practice (Butterworth and Bishop, 1995) that a system should be in place which empowers practitioners and protects patients by the regulation and promotion of good practice.

In a further drive from the DoH, the lead Nursing Officer, in collaboration with the *Nursing Times*, raised the profile of clinical supervision with practising nurses and health visitors (Bishop, 1994) and developed, in conjunction with the Trust Nurse Executives, a three-point plan in which a national workshop for Trust Nurse Executives, a national conference for the profession and a multisite evaluation research project were proposed. The two conferences were held and have been reported upon (NHS Executive 1994, 1995), the multisite evaluation project was completed in 1997 (Butterworth *et al.*, 1997).

In its most recent update on work by the professions (DoH, 1995a), commenting on the progress on target 10 of *Vision for the Future* (DoH, 1993), the NHSE suggests that:

> National initiatives which lead to improved clinical supervision, developing professional consensus on the key elements of clinical supervision and ensuring consistency with UKCC guidance should inform developments at local level. Improved understanding of the cost benefits of clinical supervision will need to be developed between purchasers and providers and a nurse or health visitor could be seconded to carry out the necessary developmental work.

The UKCC itself has issued a statement for professional guidance on clinical supervision (UKCC, 1996).

It is becoming possible to identify some evaluation techniques that can assist practitioners, purchasers and providers to assess the utility and usefulness of clinical supervision and its impact on the workforce. The following matters are seen as important in auditing and monitoring clinical supervision (Butterworth and Faugier, 1994):

- defining and agreeing the agencies' ground rules;
- devising and monitoring the agencies' plan for implementing and sustaining clinical supervision;
- looking at the provision of education and development;
- monitoring and maintaining a list of supervisors;
- deciding on a mechanism for evaluation.

Audit and evaluation

Trust Nurse Executives (NHS Executive, 1994) have suggested that it may be possible to audit clinical supervision through existing mechanisms, such as rates of sickness and absence, staff satisfaction scales, the number of patient complaints, the retention and recruitment of staff and critical incident maps. However, it is recognised that more sophisticated tools must be developed, and the recently published national study (Butterworth *et al.*, 1997) is a first collaborative attempt to develop this work further.

Using the component elements of clinical supervision as suggested by Proctor (1991), it is possible to offer the first steps in an evaluation strategy. These first steps seek to evaluate the core principle of clinical supervision, that of supporting staff. Progressively, work should also seek to link clinical supervision to clinical outcomes.

1 *The normative component* (organisational and quality control issues). By examining data already gathered for general information purposes, a Trust might find data relating to the value of clinical supervision from clinical audit, staff satisfaction scales, rates of sickness or absence and number of patient complaints. Assessment tools exist which might further inform this process (Cooper *et al.*, 1988).
2 *The restorative component* (supportive help for professionals working constantly with stress and distress). Stress, personal well-being and support can be determined from a series of reputable survey instruments (Maslach and Jackson, 1986; Goldberg and Williams, 1988; Harris, 1989; Brown *et al.*, 1995; De Villiers *et al.*, 1995), and their use in mental health nursing has been reported elsewhere (Carson *et al.*, 1995).

3   *The formative component* (the educative component of developing skills). It is suggested that this component might be evaluated using Trust-wide educational audits, live supervision on audio- or videotape, *post hoc* analysis or audio- or videotape recordings and *post hoc* analysis of observation notes.

Conclusion

What does the future hold for clinical supervision, and how will it progress in future years? It appears fashionable to make no progress on any new developments unless they can somehow be tied to patient-led outcomes and evidence-based practice, as though these laudable aims were achievable overnight. This is an objective to which we must all strive, but more often complex matters such as these will take considerable time to achieve and we must not reject non-evidence-based practice as being either wrong or necessarily of poor quality. It is vital to remember that absence of evidence does not necessarily equate with evidence of absence.

Equally, there is no need to apologise for actions that make staff feel supported and valued. The NHS is finding it hard to attract people into medicine and the health care professions, and, once it has got them, struggles to keep them. Part of the problem clearly rests in a need to value, support and sustain staff who work constantly with illness, disease and death and for whom dramatic organisational change has been a way of life for the past 15 years. If clinical supervision does this, it is worth our investment.

A sure sign of success for clinical supervision will be when it has become part of the cultural 'norm' for nurses and health visitors, and does not require the special attention it now receives in order to implement it in the clinical setting.

A future dream is to see any absence of clinical supervision as a curiosity; when this is so, we can be sure that its enculturation into the professions is complete.

Endnote

As this chapter is being produced for publication, the findings of the first national survey have been produced (Butterworth *et al.*, 1997). Having conducted a review of clinical supervision in 23 sites in England and Scotland, the results clearly show that clinical supervision has a measurably positive impact on the workforce; clinical supervision deals with such vital matters as clinical casework, organisational and management issues, professional development, educational support, confidence building and personal and interpersonal matters.

References

Bishop, V. 1994 Clinical supervision; questionnaire results. *Research in Practice* **90**(48): 40–2.

Brocklehurst, N.I. 1995 Developing a Model of Clinical Supervision for Community Nursing: The Case of District Nurses and HIV Disease. Unpublished MSc Thesis, University of Manchester.

Brown, D., Leary, J., Carson, J., Bartlett, H. and Fagin, L. 1995 Stress and the community mental health nurse: the development of a measure. *Journal of Psychiatric and Mental Health Nursing* **2**: 1–5.

Butterworth, T. 1988 Breaking the Boundaries: New Endeavours in Community Nursing, Inaugural Lecture, University of Manchester Department of Nursing.

Butterworth, T. 1992 Clinical supervision as an emerging idea in nursing. In: Butterworth, T. and Faugier, J. (eds) *Clinical Supervision and Mentorship in Nursing*. London: Chapman & Hall.

Butterworth, T. and Bishop, V. 1995 Identifying the characteristics of optimum practice: findings from a survey of practice experts in nursing, midwifery and health visiting. *Journal of Advanced Nursing* **22**: 24–32.

Butterworth, T. and Faugier, J. 1992 *Clinical Supervision of Mentorship in Nursing*. London: Chapman & Hall.

Butterworth, T. and Faugier, J. 1994 *Clinical Supervision in Nursing, Midwifery and Health Visiting: A Briefing Paper*. Manchester School of Nursing Studies, University of Manchester.

Butterworth, T., Bishop, V. and Carson, J. 1996 First steps towards evaluating clinical supervision in nursing and health visiting. Part 1: Theory, policy and practice development. *Journal of Clinical Nursing* **5**: 127–32.

Butterworth, T., Carson, J., White, E., Jeacock, J., Clements, A. and Bishop, V. 1997 *It Is Good to Talk. An Evaluation of Clinical Supervision and Mentorship in England and Scotland*. Manchester: University of Manchester School of Nursing and Midwifery.

Carson, J., Fagin, L. and Ritter, S. 1995 *Stress and Coping in Mental Health Nursing*. London: Chapman & Hall.

Cooper, C., Sloan, S. and Williams, S. 1988 *The Occupational Stress Indicator*. Windsor: NFER-Nelson.

Darling, L.A. 1985 What to do about toxic mentors. *Journal of Nursing Administration* **5**: 43–4.

Department of Health 1991 The Allitt Inquiry. Independent inquiry relating to deaths and injuries on the children's ward at Grantham and Kesteven General Hospital during the period February to April 1991. London: HMSO.

Department of Health 1993 *Vision for the Future*. Report of the Chief Nursing Officer. London: HMSO.

Department of Health 1994a *Clinical Supervision for the Nursing and Health Visiting Professions*. CNO Letter 94(5). London: HMSO.

Department of Health 1994 *Clinical Supervision: A Report of the Trust Nurse Executives Workshops*. Edited by Tony Butterworth and Veronica Bishop. London: NHS Executive.

Department of Health 1995a *Vision for the Future: Implementation and Evaluation 1995 and Beyond*. London: NHS Executive.

Department of Health 1995 *Clinical Supervision*. Conference proceedings from a national workshop at the National Motorcycle Museum. Birmingham: NHS Executive.

DeVilliers, N., Carson, J., Leary, J., O'Malley, P. and Dankert, A. 1997 *Stress in Ward Based Mental Health Nurses: The Development and Piloting of a New Measure* (in preparation).

Dewing, J. 1994 Report on Burford Community Hospital. In: Kohner, N. (ed.) *Clinical Supervision in Practice*. London: King's Fund Centre/Dorset: BEBC.

Dudley, M. and Butterworth, T. 1994 The costs and some benefits of clinical supervision: an initial exploration. *International Journal of Psychiatric Nursing Research* **1**(2): 34–40.

Faugier, J. and Butterworth, T. 1994 *Clinical Supervision: A Position Paper*. Manchester: School of Nursing Studies, University of Manchester.

Goldberg, D. and Williams, P. 1988 *A User's Guide to the General Health Questionnaire*. Windsor: NFER-Nelson.

Hallberg, I.R. and Norberg, A. 1993 Strain among nurses and their emotional reactions during one year of systematic clinical supervision combined with the implementation of individualized care in dementia nursing. *Journal of Advanced Nursing* **18**: 1860–75.

Harris, P. 1989 The nurse stress index. *Work and Stress* 3(4): 335–46.
Harris, L. 1994 Report on midwifery supervision in South Thames Regional Health Authority. In: Butterworth, T. and Bishop, V. (eds) *Clinical Supervision: A Report of the Trust Nurse Executives Workshops*. London: NHS Executive.
Houston, G. 1990 *Supervision and Counselling*. London: Rochester Foundation.
Ito, S. 1984 *Kangogaku Zasshi* 48(12): 1405.
Johnson, P. 1995 *The Community Services View*. In: *Clinical Supervision*. Conference Proceedings. London: NHS Executive.
Jones, A. 1997 The Blessed Experience, Clinical Supervision and Macmillan nurses. PhD Thesis. University of Manchester (in preparation).
Mahmood, N. 1994 Report on Cartmel Ward Prestwich Hospital. In: Kohner, N. (ed.) *Clinical Supervision in Practice*. London: King's Fund Centre/Dorset: BEBC.
Maslach, C. and Jackson, S. 1986 *Maslach Burnout Inventory*. California: Consulting Psychologists Press.
National Health Service Executive 1994 Conference proceeding on clinical supervision. The National Motorcycle Museum, Birmingham, 29 November.
National Health Service Executive 1995 Evaluating Clinical Supervision: Seminar evaluating the utility and impact of clinical supervision, London, 27 March.
Olbrich, C. 1985 Supervision as a possibility for nursing personal to reflect on professional behaviour and expand professional competence. *Krankenpfledge* 39(5):181–3.
Platt-Koch, L.M. 1986 Clinical supervision for psychiatric nurses. *Journal of Psychological Nursing* 26(1): 7–15.
Proctor, B. 1991 Supervision: a cooperative exercise in accountability. In: Marken, M. and Payne, M. (eds) *Enabling and Ensuring: Supervision in Practice*. Leicester: National Youth Bureau and Council for Education and Training in Youth and Community Work.
Semperingham, J. 1994 Report on Ellen Skellern Three Ward. In: Kohner, N. (ed.) *Clinical Supervision in Practice*. London: King's Fund Centre/Dorset: BEBC.
UKCC (United Kingdom Central Council for Nursing, Midwifery and Health Visiting) 1984 *Code of Professional Conduct for the Nurse, Midwife and Health Visitor*. London: UKCC.
UKCC (United Kingdom Central Council for Nursing, Midwifery and Health Visiting) 1992 *The Scope of Professional Practice*. London: UKCC.
UKCC (United Kingdom Central Council for Nursing, Midwifery and Health Visiting) 1996 *A Statement on Clinical Supervision*. London: UKCC.

Postscript: Supporting the initiative: the role of the UKCC

Sue Norman

The UKCC, as the regulatory body for nurses, midwives and health visitors, is charged with the responsibility of establishing and improving the standards of education, training and professional conduct in the interests of the public.

These standards, along with the Council's policies, establish the framework and principles of self-regulation and professional accountability. Clinical supervision, from the Council's perspective, provides the final link between the theory of accountability and the realities of practice.

Clinical supervision provides the framework by which practitioners are able to improve their clinical skills, in addition to enhancing their professional knowledge and values. It can only therefore be a benefit to the profession and, as such, is something to be supported and promoted.

This developmental process augments but does not replace formal means of educational preparation for practice. It incorporates mentorship and support but, again, does not deny the specific relevance of these concepts to the newly qualified practitioner and, importantly, extends throughout the practitioner's career. In time, it will become a part of the culture of practice, so that it is established as part of working life.

In supporting clinical supervision, the Council firmly believes that further opportunities will be created for nurses and health visitors to reflect on the quality of their practice, enabling them to effect change where necessary in a secure and professionally appropriate environment. Reflecting on practice will, without doubt, result in the therapeutic potential of nursing and health visiting practice being enhanced and further developed, and the potential for harm to the patient will, as a result, be minimised.

Even if this were the only benefit of clinical supervision, the Council would continue to support this initiative in the interest of public protection. The added benefit of increasing opportunities with which to support practitioners and facilitate further professional development makes clinical supervision a tool too good to be missed. The Council, in developing principles to contribute to the effective establishment of clinical supervision, was mindful of the need to secure an approach that would be both flexible and enabling. This flexibility has opened doors of opportunity for practitioners to be creative in their development of locally acceptable models to ensure the best possible results from their experience.

The Council has remained firm in its belief that the setting of clear ground rules and the adequate preparation of both the supervisor and supervisee are paramount to success. Evidence of the benefits of clinical supervision remain largely anecdotal, and the need for further evaluation at a local level remains if its true benefits are ever satisfactorily to be demonstrated.

Butterworth *et al.* (1997) in their evaluative study of 23 sites in England and Scotland, reported little statistical difference between test and control groups, although practitioners did state that the experience was positive. There is clearly more work to be done.

In conclusion, as stated in The Position Statement on Clinical Supervision for Nursing and Health Visiting (1996) the UKCC endorses the establishment of clinical supervision in the interest of maintaining and improving standards of care in an often uncertain and rapidly changing health and social care environment.

The UKCC commends clinical supervision to all practitioners, managers, and those involved in negotiating contracts as an important part of strategies to promote higher standards of nursing and health visiting care into the twenty-first-century, and this book will be invaluable in helping the profession to meet that challenge.

References

Butterworth, T., Carson, J., White, E., Jeacock, J., Clements, A. and Bishop, V. 1997 *It Is Good to Talk. An Evaluation of Clinical Supervision and Mentorship in England and Scotland*. Manchester: University of Manchester School of Nursing and Midwifery.
UKCC (United Kingdom Central Council for Nursing, Midwifery and Health Visiting) 1996 *The Position Statement on Clinical Supervision for Nursing and Health Visiting*, London.

Index

U.W.E.L. LEARNING RESOURCES